Praise for *The Defiant Mind*

"The importance of this superbly written book transcends occupation and knowledge of the disease, and should be read by all. Nearly 25 percent of everyone in Canada will suffer a stroke by the time they reach eighty years old, and almost everyone will be touched by it. This much-needed book fills a void in our literature by expressively taking the reader through the experience of suffering a stroke, which of course includes the physical disability, but also the cognitive, the emotional, and the experiential effects of this disease. *The Defiant Mind* is a story of survival and the continual path to recovery.

Stroke remains a disease that is misunderstood by most people in our society. The stroke patients that I have interacted with are in need of this type of book to better understand their disease even if their experiences are unique. Furthermore, the general public should welcome this entertaining, emotional and engaging book; it helps us to better understand this disease from the beginning and from the perspective of a patient. Finally, I would highly recommend *The Defiant Mind* for healthcare professionals and students to better understand the entire scope of this disease and not just the compartmentalized aspects that they are trained to treat, to better understand the variation in care that we provide, and to better understand what it is like to go through our healthcare system."

— Noreen Kamal PEng, PhD, Alberta Stroke Program (QuICR)

"I thoroughly enjoyed Ron Smith's book. I couldn't put it down. Even without a stroke, his book is an amazing, lucid, literate, informative read. And to think he did this after a debilitating stroke leaves me grasping for superlatives."

— Bruce Hunter, author of *In the Bear's House*, Toronto

"In *The Defiant Mind* recovery is a sort of miracle, the literary enterprise even more so. An outstanding read, it is an extraordinary balancing of the various elements of narrative. The shift between the outside reality and the emotional response to the terrible ordeal of stroke takes place with naturalness and total ease. An analytical, dispassionate mind finds its counterpart in a deeply compassionate spirit, and together they converge in a dominant feeling that is love — for family, humanity at large, nature — a great monument to wholeness."

— Ada Donati, poet, translator, art critic, Rome, Italy

"I finished reading *The Defiant Mind* and LOVED IT. Beautifully written by an accomplished writer and now stroke survivor making a clear point that defiance (with unconditional support) is the first step to making hope a reality."

— Jean Woo, Heart and Stroke Foundation, Research, Ottawa

▪

"The really important feature of Ron Smith's book is that it emphasizes the effect that stroke has on the whole person. Stroke changes your very essence, changing what you can do, how you think and feel, how you experience the world and who you are. Stroke affects your family who become your care-givers. Stroke affects your community. Because there is a modular functional anatomy of the brain, stroke manifestations can be protean depending upon what part of the brain is affected. Stroke treatment is progressing on all fronts — acute care, prevention and rehabilitation. Much remains to be learned but there is progress and more stroke patients are having better outcomes every year. We are also making progress on the organization of stroke care. In Canada, we are fortunate to have a health system that does, overall and by comparison to the rest of the world, provide very good stroke care."

— Michael D. Hill, MD MSc FRCPC, Calgary Stroke Program,
Dept. Clinical Neurosciences, Hotchkiss Brain Institute,
Cumming School of Medicine, University of Calgary

▪

"Brilliant. *The Defiant Mind: Living Inside a Stroke* has given me a deeper and more human insight into an area that I have always tried to persuade myself I understood. Not only does this memoir illuminate stroke at a personal level, but it also brings clarity to the essence of "health care." Its insights into the "cul-ture" of our hospitals and services are often awakening and humbling. This book should be required reading for all leaders in health care and for student therapists. The writing is evocative — I felt such sadness when I reached the end of the book. Many experiences that are impossible to imagine if you have not suffered a stroke are brought to life. The description of learning to roll in bed and pull oneself up while managing one's paralyzed arm and leg is the best I have read. Similarly, when Ron describes trying to put on his shirt and wheel his wheelchair for the first time, I felt panic and discomfort. And I was often over-whelmed by the "vulnerability of disability." But I was heartened when he "took over" his rehab and became a stronger self-advocate. This is a well-documented account of a stroke experience bundled into a poignant story of life, love, and family."

— Pam Aikman Ramsay, Provincial Director, Stroke Services BC, Vancouver

▪

"I really enjoyed *The Defiant Mind*. The book does a remarkable job of drawing attention to the challenges and gaps in the healthcare system while still illuminating the bright spots. It is a clear and eloquent account of a personal stroke story that more than anything else reminds us that behind every stroke is an individual and that every stroke recovery journey is unique."

— Stephanie Lawrence, Senior Manager, Communications, Heart and Stroke Foundation, Ottawa

"I know this may sound strange, but *The Defiant Mind* closed a gap for me . . . it allowed me to understand (and in a way come to peace with) my dad's stroke all these years later. I really enjoyed the book . . . my favourite part was when the author's granddaughter 'comes back' to him. It moved me to see her get closer again, and made me think of when I stopped looking at my dad differently. I don't know if Ron Smith meant for that to be a tipping point in his recovery for his readers, but it definitely was for me."

— Elizabeth Takac, Coordinator, Research, Heart and Stroke Foundation

"Ron Smith has written a wonderful book about surviving a stroke. *The Defiant Mind: Living Inside a Stroke* is a MUST READ for stroke survivors, their caregivers, as well as a general audience. Every year, strokes permanently disable five million people worldwide; consequently, how to treat stroke survivors has become a fundamental health issue facing us today.

I honestly thought I knew something about stroke before reading this book. I have a doctorate in Neuroscience from the UCLA Brain Research Center and do research on cardiovascular diseases. I also have experience as a caregiver. Several years ago, when my parents were visiting us, my mother suffered a massive stroke at our house two days after Christmas. Despite her age, she was a very healthy individual with normal blood pressure who kept fit by playing tennis daily. The stroke was completely unexpected and devastating for our family. Although she was hospitalized within an hour of the stroke, she died about one month later. I never gained much insight into her suffering because of her severely debilitated state. Ron's book really opened my eyes.

I started reading *The Defiant Mind* thinking it would confirm what I already knew. Nothing could have been further from the truth. We tend to judge a stroke survivor's progress by external factors, such as the gains they make in strength, or their improved ability to walk and speak. But that is only a small part of the story. Here, we have a first-hand account of the perceived inner workings of a brain scrambled by a stroke, trying to make sense of the world around it. The subtle things that those of us on the outside normally miss or think irrelevant, Ron shows to be absolutely crucial.

Ron's account of his recovery is fascinating, frustrating and powerful. How his mind goes from being decimated by oxygen deprivation during the stroke to the processes involved in trying to make new neuronal connections to understand the world is illuminating, and told from a perspective that most of us have never imagined. The resurfacing of archival memories in the author's brain from forty to fifty years ago as if they had happened yesterday is truly insightful to me, not only as a scientist but as someone who has cared for a loved one who has experienced a stroke. The frustration of not being able to communicate with family and friends, the challenges the survivor faces in the often long recovery process and the determination it takes to make a strong recovery are compelling. A captivating read, this book helps us better understand stroke from the INSIDE.

One of the ironies of my writing about *The Defiant Mind* is that I am about to take my son to the hospital to visit a thirty-five-year-old co-worker of his who suffered a stroke on the job last week. I'm having my son read Ron Smith's book as a way to understand what she is going through and to help him see how he can assist in her recovery."

— Glen Tibbits, PhD, Professor and Chair, Biomedical Physiology and Kinesiology, SFU; Canada Research Chair in Molecular Cardiac Physiology; Vice Chair of the Scientific Review Committee, Heart and Stroke Foundation of Canada

THE Defiant MIND

OTHER BOOKS BY
RON SMITH

Seasonal (1984)

A Buddha Named Baudelaire (1988)

Enchantment and Other Demons (1995)

The Last Time We Talked (1996)

What Men Know About Women (1999)

Arabesque e altre poesie
(Italian translation by Ada Donati, 2002)

Elf the Eagle (2007)

Kid Dynamite: The Gerry James Story (2011)

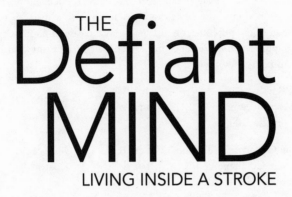

THE
Defiant
MIND

LIVING INSIDE A STROKE

RON SMITH

RONSDALE PRESS

RONSDALE PRESS
3350 West 21st Avenue, Vancouver, BC, Canada V6S 1G7
www.ronsdalepress.com

Typesetting: Julie Cochrane, in Bembo 12 pt on 16
Cover Design: Julie Cochrane
Cover Art: Jack Shadbolt, "Bursting Orb"
Paper: Ancient Forest Friendly "55 lb Offset Natural" (FSC) —
    100% post-consumer waste, totally chlorine-free and acid-free

Ronsdale Press wishes to thank the following for their support of its publishing program: the Canada Council for the Arts, the Government of Canada through the Canada Book Fund, the British Columbia Arts Council, and the Province of British Columbia through the British Columbia Book Publishing Tax Credit program.

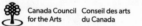   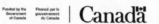

Library and Archives Canada Cataloguing in Publication

Smith, Ron, 1943 August 7–, author
   The defiant mind: living inside a stroke / Ron Smith. — First edition.

Includes bibliographical references.
Issued in print and electronic formats.
ISBN 978-1-55380-480-2 (hardback) / ISBN 978-1-55380-464-2 (paperback)
ISBN 978-1-55380-465-9 (ebook) / ISBN 978-1-55380-466-6 (pdf)

   1. Smith, Ron, 1943 August 7–. 2. Cerebrovascular disease — Popular works. 3. Cerebrovascular disease — Patients — Biography. I. Title.

RC388.5.S65 2016   616.8'1   C2016-902099-1   C2016-902100-9

At Ronsdale Press we are committed to protecting the environment. To this end we are working with Canopy and printers to phase out our use of paper produced from ancient forests. This book is one step towards that goal.

Printed in Canada by Friesens, Manitoba

For Pat, Nicole and Owen

And for Frances Kern

"Rabbit's clever," said Pooh thoughtfully.

"Yes," said Piglet, "Rabbit's clever."

"And he has Brain."

"Yes," said Piglet, "Rabbit has Brain."

There was a long silence.

"I suppose," said Pooh, "that that's why he never understands anything."

— A.A. Milne, *Winnie-the-Pooh*

"I'm not lost for I know where I am. But however, where I am may be lost."

— A.A. Milne, *Winnie-the-Pooh*

CONTENTS

*Every forty seconds someone
in North America suffers a stroke.*

*Every four minutes someone in
North America dies from a stroke.*

*Stroke is the leading cause of disability
in North America.*

The Defiant Mind: Living Inside a Stroke took me over a year and a half
to write, pecking one letter at a time with the index finger on my
left hand. Eventually I learned to use my thumb to hit the space bar.
This process was by no means as slow as signalling each letter of each
word by blinking one eye, as was Jean-Dominique Bauby's method
of dictation when he composed his exquisite *The Diving-Bell and the
Butterfly.* Yet, compared to my typing eighty words a minute prior to
my stroke, I lumbered along writing this book, like the tortoise in
Aesop's fable. I was determined to win the race, but my lone finger had
difficulty keeping up with the pace of my thoughts. Those thoughts
ran ahead like the hare, who stopped, every so often, to nap. Meanwhile, my finger poked and plodded along, and I finally crossed the
finish line, my thoughts and finger arriving at pretty much the
same time.

The book is completed, even though my right hand and arm, foot and leg still suffer from the effects of spasticity. And even though, as far as I know, I've emerged a somewhat altered person. Later, much later in my recovery, an internist told me that the difference between a heart attack and a stroke is that after a heart attack you at least know who you are.

My story begins with the first hint that something unusual was happening to me, on a day that began like any other and ended with my body and brain suffering a frontal assault of such magnitude that I was left severely disabled. The actual attack lasted for several hours, perhaps days. No one knew for sure how long my brain was under siege or how many brain cells had been destroyed. The initial CT scan taken the evening I ended up in hospital showed nothing, but a few days later, after another image was taken, the damage was writ large for everyone to see. I now had the road map for the attack on my brain stem, but no one seemed able or willing to explain why it had happened.

As is the case with all strokes, mine was haphazard and unique.

Perhaps the most frightening thing for me was that I was rapidly losing contact with the world I knew. Suddenly nothing made sense anymore. On the one hand, I wondered why all the fuss; on the other, I knew I needed help.

But what would help?

And who?

To exercise my brain and in the hope of finding out what had happened to me, I spent a considerable part of the second half of my first year of rehab reading books about the brain and a few about brain attacks suffered by other stroke survivors, including books by Jill Bolte Taylor, Bonnie Sherr Kline, Robert McCrum, as well as Jean-Dominique Bauby. Each one gave a disturbing if not chilling account of their stroke. They talked about the loss of cognitive powers, about being "locked in" (like Stephen Hawking with his ALS), about being handicapped, about the stress put on relationships, especially family and marriage. And about the triumph of love and the power of the "will to be" as keys to the effectiveness of the lengthy rehabilitation process.

Their stories helped to show me some ways to recovery, and yet something important seemed to be missing from their accounts. No one discussed the role of mind and memory in reasserting a sense of self. Despite the huge pummelling I had taken, I began to realize that my fragments of memory confirmed not only "who I was" but gave me the "will to be."

Another thing, their strokes were hemorrhagic — a bleed in the brain — the rarest form of stroke, while mine was ischemic — a clot or blockage in the brain — which is the most common type of stroke, accounting for approximately 82 to 87 percent of strokes.

One key point to know when reading this account: In the early days after my stroke, I lost my ability to forget. All the protective defences I had learned since childhood were destroyed. I was bombarded by the pandemonium of sounds, images, memories and emotions that flood our brains at every moment of our daily lives. At first I didn't know how to cope with this explosion of sensations and thoughts, but slowly I learned to live again through my memories. As I lay in my hospital bed, memory became my salvation.

As the world about me became more turbulent, I drew more heavily on my past. My hunger pains in the hospital triggered memories of nearly starving in my youth and caused me to relive a trip I took to Spain in the winter of 1964/1965. By recalling how I dealt with events that had dislocated me then — allowing me to survive — I found a way of relocating myself in the "now" and reclaiming who I was.

My stroke account moves in and out of past and present — between a past in which I lived amongst people inhabiting far-away lands who spoke in foreign tongues, and a present in which I lived amongst people who occupied a world where I now felt like a foreigner and with whom I struggled to communicate with my new thick and unresponsive tongue. The travel memories in my book, which serve as a metaphor for the recovery of my self, recount the ways I found of saying, "I am alive and I am still thinking."

When I was able to stay awake, my brain was hyperactive, flooded with ideas and impressions, to the point where I began to feel over-whelmed. When I was on the edge of sleep and feeling under siege, I asked myself:

How am I to avoid being overwhelmed?

How might I find my way back?

How might I rediscover my old self?

From my perspective, I ended up living inside the stroke. I was no longer in the everyday walkabout world as a functioning member of society. In the following pages I have attempted to provide a day-by-day account of what was happening to me, and what I learned that might help in future therapeutic practice. I describe the process by which my memories helped me to reassert who I was and gave me the will to continue. At times the endeavour was comical, at times fiercely depersonalizing.

I soon understood that I could either give in to the despair that haunts many stroke patients or figure out a way to rebuild all those bridges in the brain that define who I am. I knew I had to escape from the bottle of voices and ideas that threatened to overwhelm me. I needed to rediscover the regulator or "governor" that keeps the traffic in the brain organized and at speed. Otherwise chaos would set in.

Since my stroke, as part of my self-directed therapy, I have read widely about brain research. The ability of the brain to recreate or modify its structure is the foundation of the important and exciting work now being done on what is referred to as brain plasticity.

Therein, I believe, lies the promise of reconnecting and reformatting — in essence, healing — the traumatized brain.

Months into recovery when I was doing research on strokes and was particularly interested in researching the brain, I dipped into A.A. Milne's *The World of Pooh*, which seemed to sum up perfectly what a stroke entailed for the survivor and what it meant to many of the people a stroke survivor was likely to meet. A common response to someone who has suffered a stroke is that they no longer have a functioning brain and, if they do, it's lost and they're elsewhere. I suddenly found myself being treated like a curiosity at best, as an "untouchable" at worst. I felt I needed to keep saying, "I'm not a stranger, and I'm not a cabbage, I have eyes and, like Rabbit, I have brain."

My recovery continues, and I'm optimistic that one day I will regain at least 80 percent of my previous mobility. A whole community of people has contributed to my recovery: friends, neighbours, family, nurses, doctors, therapists.

Over the course of two years I learned that many health professionals make a puzzling and disturbing separation between the body and the brain. While therapists and doctors helped with my physical recovery, I learned that the restoration of my cognitive "being" was up to me. No one seemed interested in what was happening inside my brain. No one seemed interested in my "subjective" thoughts — experiences which J. Allan Hobson (who himself suffered a stroke fourteen years ago and is professor emeritus of the Harvard Medical School) argues should be central to stroke research and understanding.

Each stroke event is unique because each brain is unique. This is the mantra which is continually repeated by health professionals, but is too often ignored in treatment. My book advocates for a greater focus on the brain in stroke assessment and recovery, and for placing a much greater importance on the subjective, anecdotal accounts of stroke survivors.

"Listen," each stroke survivor should demand, "I need to be heard."

At its heart, *The Defiant Mind: Living Inside a Stroke* is a book about the wonder that is the human brain, both before it has been damaged and after, when it's struggling to pick up the pieces and make some sense of the muddle it has become — the jigsaw puzzle of scattered recollections, unidentifiable objects, inexplicable emotions, impenetrable ideas. Unfortunately, as our population ages, more and more people are going to experience strokes, although it is important to note that strokes hit at any age, from infants to teenagers to young and middle-aged adults. Disturbingly, the Heart and Stroke Foundation tells us, ". . . there has been an increase in strokes among people under sixty-five and an increase in all stroke risk factors for younger adults."

At a time when the medical profession is bracing itself for an assault on the health system, health care professionals are actively looking for ways to make their interventions more patient focused. For this reason, months after I suffered my stroke, I decided I would write the story of my brain attack, giving an inside-out view of stroke and, more importantly, showing everyone that *recovery is possible*. Since many stroke victims cannot speak for themselves, my goal has been to write a book that provides a voice for victims, and gives insight and encouragement to families, friends, caregivers, medical professionals and the general reader by demonstrating that *rabbit* (that would be me and my fellow stroke survivors) truly *has brain*.

ONE

Haphazard: In Denial

Imagine. Imagine you suddenly see the world disappearing down a tunnel. Darkness surrounds a diminishing circle of light as it recedes into the distance. Light is leaving you.

You turn to your partner of forty-four years and say, "I'm dying. Please get help. Quickly. Please."

You feel an urgency that you can't quite transmit through your voice, although she appears to understand. You speak softly, your sense of desperation a mere whisper. All energy has left you. Your limbs feel limp, your body sags into itself like a bean bag. You begin to slide off the front edge of your chair. Suddenly. Involuntarily. You are in slow-motion free fall. Perhaps it's resignation. Whatever happens will happen. There seems to be an inevitability about this event that you don't comprehend but that you curiously accept. Your body and spirit have been deflated in an inexplicable way. You are experiencing a mystery. And you are terrified.

You have heard stories before from people who claim to have travelled to the "other side," stories about tunnels and light, but they have always struck you as fairy tales or hallucinations brought on by fear. The mind is a gifted field of play. But this is real, as real as your partner running towards the nursing station and crying out for help.

How distant her voice sounds.

Never have you been so scared.

The one thing you know at that moment is that you have no control over your destiny. You are at the mercy of everything that surrounds you: patients, a buggy, chairs, stretchers, a phone ringing, movement, voices, a baby crying, a couple looking at you oddly from across the room, and the disappearing light.

This is what happened to me at about ten o'clock on the evening of November 19, 2012, in the waiting room of emergency at the Nanaimo Regional General Hospital.

But that is not where my story begins. My stroke story. Here's how events unfolded.

Earlier that day, just before noon, I stood in the doorway of the bathroom in our Nanoose Bay home watching my wife making final preparations to go out for lunch with a group of friends. I had spent the morning writing or editing. I don't remember which. Now I was watching her, watching with the same pleasure I have always received from seeing the final transformation she makes when she "puts her face on." To be honest, I don't see too much of a difference. I think she's quite tasty, face on or face off, but there is something exquisite and magical in the ritual of a woman putting on makeup.

As I leaned against the door jamb, saying my customary goodbyes, telling her to enjoy herself and taking in an eyeful of the woman I have loved for close to half a century, I felt a bit odd. Not in response to anything she was doing, but inside myself. I didn't feel nauseated or faint, simply odd. Perhaps a bit weak. Otherwise there was nothing out of the ordinary that a brief lie down wouldn't cure.

So I bid my wife *au revoir* and sprawled out on the bed. As soon as my head hit the pillow, I drifted into sleep. I have no other recollections from that time, although I was surprised to discover when I awoke that two hours had passed. I'm fond of naps. This is often when I do my most productive thinking, but napping for this length of time was extreme.

I staggered to my feet, stretched and thought, I've got to get some work done. I'm a charter member of the generation that feels guilty if I haven't made my daily contribution to the sweat pool. Or spent a couple of brain cells on an idea that hopefully seemed clever. The Protestant work ethic has me firmly in grasp.

I made my way to my study, sat down in front of my computer to work and immediately noticed my right hand was crawling over the keys. My left hand was dancing in step to my thoughts but my right hand was sluggish; in fact, it required all my concentration to move each finger. They appeared to have a will of their own. They looked and behaved like lobster claws, moving in slow motion. I paused. This was definitely strange. I remember examining the keyboard and thinking somehow it would reveal an answer to what was going on. Without much forethought I typed "stroke" into Google. I'm not sure why I did this, although for some time I had developed the habit of searching the Web for possible explanations for the increasingly peculiar things my body was doing in response to ageing. The Internet was turning me into a hypochondriac. I can't tell you why I chose "stroke" on this occasion and not heart attack or some other more exotic ailment such as Lyme disease or mad cow disease.

Several sites popped up on the screen, each containing a list of common symptoms for someone having a stroke:

- Sudden numbness or weakness of face, arms or legs — especially on one side of the body.
- Sudden confusion, trouble speaking or understanding.
- Sudden trouble seeing in one or both eyes.

■ Sudden trouble walking, dizziness, and/or loss of balance or coordination.

■ Sudden severe headache with no known cause.

Some sites recommended three simple tests I could perform to ascertain if I were having a stroke:

■ Can you raise your arms and keep them up?

■ Can you smile?

■ Can you repeat a simple sentence?

I passed the tests with flying colours. I lifted my arms above my head, smiled, made up a sentence to repeat and repeated it. Flawlessly. Happily, I told myself, you're not having a stroke. As far as I could figure out, none of the symptoms applied to my situation.

I was relieved, of course, and immediately in denial. I was to learn that denial is an all-too-common response to having a stroke. In addition to that, I'm male and . . . well, you know the story. Perhaps I felt the list of symptoms was too vague. Because "inability to type" didn't appear on the list, I reasoned my problem was annoying, uncomfortable and worrisome, but definitely did not qualify as a signal for something as serious as a stroke. But, and this is a huge "but," if I had thought about the list of symptoms, I would have recognized that number one on the list fit what was happening to me to a T. Undoubtedly my intuition to type "stroke" into the search engine of my computer was way ahead of my powers of logic, of my ability to observe and reason.

Clearly one part of one side of my body was weak. The first sign of a symptom was present. A simple signal, yes, but one I was more than happy to ignore or rationalize away as anything but a stroke. After all, I didn't want to have a stroke. Who does? We belong to a culture of invulnerability, especially the male side of the species, and to admit to an ache or pain or, God forbid, an illness, is a sign of weakness. To compound the problem of my defiance, I have to confess here and now, I really knew very, very little about what it is to have a stroke and what the actual word means, in spite of the vigorous attempts by various organizations to warn us about what I can now testify is a massive assault on the brain and body, mentally, physically and spiritually.

I should have been forewarned!

Figuring that I had done my due diligence and still feeling "poorly," I went back to bed. I felt okay as long as I was at rest and prone. (Wow, was that a portent of things to come!) By now I think I had reduced my symptoms to that catch-all illness, the flu. I had the flu, that was it. There was a certain comfort in settling on this familiar "bug," no matter how vague and expansive I was making the symptoms. For the most part, I was satisfied with this diagnosis, but the image of my uncooperative hand and fingers still nagged at the back of my mind. And I still felt "odd," a feeling for which I lacked an adequate description — I was struggling here because I had never felt this way before — but if I were honest, I would have to confess that feeling "odd" felt a lot like "light-headed."

Bingo! A second symptom which I chose to ignore had reared its ugly head. I had no desire to translate my word "light-headed" into dizziness or lack of coordination. As far as I was concerned my "light-headedness" was, well, one of those things associated with the flu. Along with upset stomach, a sniffle and so on.

I was now forewarned and still in denial.

The biggest challenge confronting all those organizations who vigilantly, desperately, try to alert us to the symptoms of a stroke is that every stroke is haphazard and unique, often in ways that are quite subtle. Trying to generalize and then broadcast those symptoms to an often ill-informed and unreceptive public is incredibly difficult.

After all, the majority of us are healthy, and that is, understandably, how we want to continue to think about and imagine ourselves.

I have known a few stroke survivors (I used to think of them as victims), but I had never seriously questioned what that meant. I never bothered with a follow-up inquiry. I would express my sympathy and get on with my life, as callous as that now sounds. I didn't know how their stroke had affected them, nor did I have a clue about the challenges they faced in recovery. I was admittedly ignorant, blissfully so. Like most people, I lived in my bubble of wellness.

And, that afternoon, I embraced my ignorance by going back to bed.

My rest was fitful as the image of my fingers lumbering about the keyboard like five drunken puppets that had had their strings cut kept staggering into my consciousness. I wanted to get up and go back to work, but, frankly, I felt better lying down.

At about four o'clock I heard my wife open and close the back door. I could hear her move about the house in search of me. When she entered the bedroom, she remarked:

"You're still in bed!"

"Yes," was the only answer I could muster.

"Are you still feeling poorly?"

"Yes."

"Do you think we should head into emergency?"

"No," I insisted. "I've probably got the flu. I'd be wasting their time and resources. Besides, they might want to keep me in, and I'm not keen to spend a night in hospital."

Aha, I had finally revealed another part of the truth behind my refusal to make the half-hour drive into town.

"Who is keen?" she asked. I could tell my wife was annoyed with my response.

From the time she arrived home, she was fairly relentless about my going into emergency.

"What harm can it do?" she said, her tone somewhat accusatory, these her final words on the subject, at least for the moment.

She busied herself moving various things around the kitchen, "tidying up" she called it. Her back stiffened, each object set on the counter, each drawer closed, coming to rest a little more forcefully and louder than usual. No more words were spoken.

Another hour passed and we continued to dither. Yet I still felt "odd" and a bit nervous that my symptoms persisted. Finally she suggested we phone a friend who had recently experienced a TIA (transient ischemic attack or warning stroke), which is when the symptoms last only a short time, less than an hour. Of course, our friend was not a medical person, and even if she were, how would she know what was happening to me from a description given over the phone? She couldn't! But for some reason and, thankfully, her recent event leant her opinion some authority.

When Pat called her, Marg said: "If you think there is even the slightest chance he is having a stroke, get your butt into emergency!"

Though not dragged kicking and screaming, I was a reluctant passenger as my wife pulled our car out of the driveway and headed for the hospital. Secretly, I have to admit, I was somewhat relieved.

Subsequently I have learned that there were two things wrong with my response. First, my body was speaking to me, but I was refusing to hear the message. Okay, I know my body better than anyone else, but that does not equip me with the skills to make a correct diagnosis of sudden changes in my body's behaviour. I want my doctors and nurses to listen to me and then weigh that information in combination with their vast experience. Any medical person worthy of their stethoscope needs to weigh anecdotal evidence against their years of training and practical knowledge. Fortunately this happened for me when I finally reached the emergency room and the doctor on duty.

And second, the advice I had read on all the stroke-related websites stated emphatically, if any of the symptoms of a stroke persist, call 9-1-1. Stupidly and stubbornly, I didn't heed this advice.

I can't emphasize how important this often-ignored suggestion is.

Put simply, immediate attention could save your life! Had I used common sense I could have prevented myself years of unnecessary grief. If you arrive at emergency in an ambulance, you are undoubtedly in knowledgeable hands and, more importantly, you will likely shoot to the front of the queue, especially if there is the slightest chance you are having a stroke. You will probably receive a CAT scan or "CT of the head" more quickly, which will tell medical staff whether or not you are having an ischemic (an abrupt blockage of arteries leading to the brain) or hemorrhagic (bleeding into the brain tissue when a blood vessel bursts) stroke. And if it is an ischemic stroke you are having, there are drugs that can be administered — these medications are time sensitive and must be administered within approximately four and a half hours of symptom onset — that will break up the clot and perhaps lessen the extent of the brain damage you will suffer. Or a quick diagnosis could save your life.

Around 20 percent of strokes suffered in North America and Europe are fatal. Worldwide, according to the World Health Organization, that figure jumps to 33 percent, bad odds by any reckoning. Even though the survival rate has improved over the past few years, I'd like to see those odds improved.

My wife pulled up to the doors of emergency around seven in the evening. She dropped me off while she went to park the car. With the aid of my walking stick, a gift she had given me the previous summer on a visit to Dawson City and the Top of the World Highway, I managed to weave my way to reception. I was feeling increasingly unsteady. My legs felt quite feeble, almost wobbly. I sat down to await my turn at the admittance desk. Ahead of me was a young man with a nasty-looking arm wound. Had he been in a knife fight or was the gash the result of a silly accident? He took one look at me and gestured that I go to the desk first. He seemed to have a better sense of my plight than I did. Needless to say I was grateful.

As my wife (she had now joined me) and I filled in the necessary paperwork and my medical card was swiped into the system, the receptionist peppered us with questions. While I still denied that I was having a stroke, my wife placed it at the top of her list of possibilities. In fact, I think it may have been the only concern on her list. The receptionist immediately shifted her questions to my wife. What had she noticed that led her to this conclusion? And so on.

Meanwhile, I was becoming slightly impatient, which in turn pumped adrenalin throughout my body; I suddenly felt much perkier and a little more defiant. Likely my blood pressure also shot up a few points! I was determined to prove everyone wrong. I had the flu, pure and simple. My case was not unique and did not warrant special attention. So much for self-awareness.

After checking in, Pat and I took seats in the emergency waiting room, amongst a hodgepodge of characters: young and old, male and female, some relaxed, some clearly uncomfortable. One scruffy older man, probably younger than me, kept looking at me with a side glance and then finally leaned over and said:

"I've been admiring your walking stick."

I did not want his attention and felt a bit annoyed that he had invaded my space. Quickly I muttered, "Oh! Well, yes, thank you." He was just trying to be friendly, but I was in a funk.

"Do you mind if I have a look?"

I handed him the stick, simultaneously inhaling a powerful whiff of booze. He rotated it with his fingers while exclaiming, "Yes, yes, a fine stick. Nicely turned out. The knob is a thoughtful touch. Easy to grip and a friendly feel. Just the right size for the palm of the hand. Do you know what kind of wood it is?"

I hadn't a clue and shook my head. I wondered how someone could find so much to say about a crooked length of wood. A bowed branch cut from a tree. But, no, he was right; my walking stick was a beautiful object. Round and smooth, ringed by ridges that looked as though they had been carefully carved by a master craftsman. I remember wondering why I was finding it so difficult to be charitable. The calm that surrounded me seemed only to feed my fury.

Shortly thereafter a casually dressed man, sleeves rolled up, collar open, called out my name and gestured towards one of the examining rooms. I glanced at the clock; it was just short of nine. At last, I thought, we can put an end to this nonsense. He looked a reasonable man.

The doctor asked me to take a seat on the examining table, one of those stuffed vinyl-covered benches divided into sections so your body can be shifted to different heights for closer and more comfortable probing.

For the moment he simply asked me to sit facing him. He wanted to know why I was in emergency. I immediately launched into a somewhat dismissive explanation of my wife's concern that I might be suffering a stroke. My hands threw out this and that, as if I were feeding bread crumbs to pigeons in the park. He stopped me. He said he would like a detailed account of what had been happening to me from the time I first felt "odd."

"Take your time, every detail is important, no matter how insignificant you might think it is," he told me.

I then recounted as much as I could remember of my day. Thoroughly. I was proud of my memory. Then he told me he would like to perform a number of simple tests.

"Do you mind?"

"No, of course not. Anything to resolve the matter once and for all."

Besides, by now I was both curious and worried.

I don't recall the full battery of tests but they seemed comprehensive enough. He asked me to touch the end of my nose with the index finger of each hand. He asked me to keep my head still and follow his index finger with my eyes only as it moved through space. He asked me to count backwards by sevens. He had me squeeze two of his fingers with each hand. He removed my shoes and socks and tested each of my feet for feeling. He tested my reflexes and asked me questions to determine if my cognitive abilities had been compromised in any way.

I was ecstatic! He was unable to stump me. Everything appeared to be functioning normally. I had passed every test he had thrown at me.

I thought: I'm going home to sleep in my own bed! Just as I predicted, I'm as healthy as the proverbial horse. Hallelujah.

What I had been experiencing was just a hiccup, some temporary malfunction of my wiring or plumbing.

"I'd like to keep you in for observation," he said.

My jaw must have dropped just short of the floor. I remember feeling a wedge of panic insert itself between jubilation and disbelief.

"Why?" I asked. "Didn't I just pass all of your tests? I did much the same thing at home in response to the stroke sites," I pointed out. "I would rather spend the night in the comfort of my own bed. This is why I didn't want to come here in the first place. I knew this would happen."

It was as though I had been tricked by sleight of hand.

I was adamant. There was no way I was going to spend the night in a hospital bed. Now I sounded as though I were blaming him for my being there. All I could do was stare at him, totally dumbfounded. I felt like the kid caught climbing the neighbour's apple tree.

"Five nights. It will be for five nights," he told me.

"Five nights," I exclaimed, "you've got to be kidding?"

"No, I wouldn't kid you about a matter this serious. And, yes, you did pass all of the tests."

He was trying to slip the rug out from under me. I felt as though some unspoken promise or contract had been broken.

"No," I said, trying to construct an argument that would see me safely on my way. "No, I don't think so. I'm not at all excited about spending the best part of a week in a hospital room. A room I'll probably have to share with someone who is seriously ill. I don't like that prospect. As you say, I passed all of your tests and I don't see the benefit."

In retrospect, the extent and degree of my denial was embarrassing. Logic had totally abandoned me. I had sought this man's advice, admittedly somewhat against my will, and he was giving me his informed opinion. I sensed he was genuinely concerned about me, but that didn't seem to matter. I was determined to have my way and make my escape.

He was to tell me later that even though I had passed his tests, there was something worrying in my anecdotal account of events and feelings that had, in his mind, set off alarm bells. And I thank my lucky stars it did. If I had persuaded him to release me, there is no doubt I would not be here today.

"It's up to you," he said gently and rather too solemnly, "but we could be talking about your life here. I think you might be having what we call a stuttering stroke."

That last comment floored me. Stroke! It finally registered with me that he thought I was having a stroke. He agreed with Pat.

He gave me a moment to digest this thought.

"A stuttering stroke is a stroke that happens over several hours, perhaps even several days. You've likely had a number of mini-strokes throughout the day, since noon, when you first felt weak and 'flu-ish.' If that's the case, the likelihood of being struck by a much larger stroke is very probable."

"You mean I should have come into emergency earlier?"

"Probably yes, although with this sort of stroke I'm not sure it would have made too much of a difference. Being in the hospital has obvious advantages."

"So you're not sure," I continued to argue. "I might be fine? I might return home and sleep peacefully in my own bed? With no further occurrence?"

"Possibly, but I don't think so, and I don't think that would be wise. Predicting strokes is not an exact science. I can't over-emphasize the risks."

Had he been a weaker man he would have despaired at my stubbornness. My defiance. Or simply let me go. We had come to an impasse. He watched me calmly; I looked around the room, waiting him out. Like a poker player, bluffing. He refused to give up on me. Finally we made eye contact.

"Okay," I said. "I guess you're right."

And to be honest, I *knew* he was.

Without a hint of exaggeration I owe my life to my wife, Pat, who kept insisting I go into emergency, and to this soft-spoken, unassuming emergency doctor who, first of all, listened to me and then had the strength of will as a human being and belief in his own skills as a healer to insist I remain in hospital for observation.

As we stepped out of the examination room, he asked if anyone had accompanied me to the hospital.

"My wife," I said. "You remember, she's the one who got me into this mess."

I laughed, the sort of laugh you resort to when your thoughts are at odds with the truth.

He ignored my rather sad attempt at irony, my last-ditch attempt to paint a different outcome to this little episode, an outcome that better suited my wishes. One that confirmed I was healthy even though I knew that for years I'd been neglecting my body. I'd recently had major back surgery and I was overweight. I did far too much sitting and too much eating, a simple recipe for heart attack or stroke. As pathetic as it now seems, at least I had that much awareness.

"Good. I'd like to talk to her," he said.

Pat joined us and the good doctor then summarized the highlights of our interview and examination. She nodded as he explained his diagnosis, in particular the nature of a stuttering stroke. Meanwhile, my thoughts drifted beyond the hushed busyness of the emergency area to a dazed review of the day's events. The ledger for my side of the argument looked pretty bleak, filled mostly with red ink. I felt nervous because deep down I instinctively knew there was a good chance the doctor was right. I worried that I really was not as healthy as I pretended to be. What if he were right?

As they finished their conversation, I looked around the room. Everyone appeared to be in a "holding pattern." Not a person had moved since I'd gone in for my consultation, although a few people had joined the ranks of those waiting. My friend with a passion for walking sticks waved and smiled at me.

"I've packed his toiletries and dressing gown, which should be enough for the night," Pat mentioned. "I'll bring in whatever else is needed tomorrow." She took my hand and held it. "I'm pleased you've talked some sense into him. Thank you, Doctor."

The doctor then told us to take our seats back in the waiting room and someone would be along for me as soon as they had a free bed.

I thanked him for his concern and advice, albeit without the conviction I would later come to know he deserved.

Then as we walked across the room, I glanced at Pat and said, as I shifted my eyes upwards, "Does someone have to depart before they have a spare bed?"

She shook her head.

I was not in a good mood. While this new wing of the hospital was fresh, bright, and upbeat, almost architecturally interesting, with water cascading down one wall and every modern convenience at hand, all I could see was a grimness to the place that all institutions somehow manage to impart. Perhaps it was the sense of efficiency and singular purpose that deprived the place of humanity when it was most needed. Or perhaps in this instance I was being unkind and transferring my own unreasonable fear and impatience onto my surroundings.

We took seats at the far side of the room, this time at a right angle to a younger couple engrossed in one of those animated conversations that has a curious restraint to it, like shadowboxing inside a phone booth. They showed not the slightest interest in my walking stick, which I used to prop up my chin and from which vantage point I now stared out into space.

Pat sat quietly beside me working on a crossword puzzle, something I knew she did when she wanted to be alone with her thoughts. Out of contact with the world. This had to be an ordeal for her, especially the uncertainty.

Glancing around the room, I felt both agitated and lost, in a space that was confining and that confirmed none of my usual impressions of the world. There were no books or paintings or plants; the only voice was a baby's, the only other sound the wheeze of a respirator.

At that moment, when I should have felt gratitude, the prospect of spending a week in hospital looked to me more like a form of incarceration. I was going to serve a sentence for serious bodily neglect. Worst of all, one that was self-inflicted!

Yes, I thought, I'm going to be a prisoner.

Prisons, I speculated, where sense deprivation is the rule, are similar to hospitals. Run by rules and regulations. Otherwise how else to keep mobs of malcontents, crooks, murderers and social misfits under control? The problem these days, though, I mused, is that prisons are filled with people who need psychiatric help and a healthy dose of tolerance and compassion, not system shutdown.

My mind wandered like a gypsy, happily seeking shelter in any byway of thought that protected me from facing the stubborn reality that there was a reason why I was waiting in the emergency room of a hospital.

What strange musings to be having, I thought. I watched a young couple fretting over their baby. It wouldn't stop crying, which by now I was sure bothered them more than what had brought them to emergency in the first place. I wanted to help them, but I was having enough difficulty containing my own sense of panic.

For some reason, the modern and crisp lines of the waiting room, the total functionality of it, brought to mind a visit I had once made to King's College Chapel, Cambridge, during the early 1960s.

On a cold mid-November day, the same time of year, with the place to myself, I was sitting near the altar admiring a Rubens triptych that was later to be defaced with the initials "I" "R" "A." No one ever determined who the vandals were, although "who" seemed obvious to me from the moment I read about it. Hadn't they left behind a pretty clear calling card?

As I studied the painting, the organ pipes burst into life, filling that beautiful Gothic space with an exquisite sound. Not with the expected choral or church music but with jazz, a sound so at odds with those soaring arches that time collapsed in on itself. Sound bounded between the stone walls and filled the heart. As the organist lost himself in his impromptu concert, I was treated to one of the most unforgettable musical moments of my life. What acoustics! Talk about heavenly! When a hush finally fell upon the place, I got up to leave. At the exit I came face to face with the musician himself as he descended the stairs from the organ loft. Obviously he hadn't seen me at the front of the church; this had been intended as a solo performance in every sense of the word. He flushed a lovely shade of crimson before I thanked him for an amazing and shared hour of bliss. Hearing my words, he looked relieved, smiled and thanked me.

Why I remembered this event at that moment in the newly completed waiting room of a hospital half a world away and fifty years later, I have no idea. Perhaps it had something to do with my interest in how we fit into space or in how space surrounds us. And the effect those spaces have on us and on our health. Two more dissimilar buildings and experiences I couldn't begin to envision.

I felt uneasy being put on hold. Nervous. I wanted to be checked in, officially. I wanted them, whoever "they" were, to get on with the blood tests and scans that would reveal what was causing me to feel "odd."

I fussed and squirmed in my seat. I remember trying to find a comfortable way to sit, something I suddenly found extremely hard to do.

Then it happened.

Just like that.

With no warning.

None.

The light started to disappear. Not fade, but close in on itself. Into a tunnel.

Soon there would be no light, I could sense that. There would be an absence. Of everything. Of everyone. Of Pat.

I remember saying, "I'm dying," and asking her to go for help.

Dead. I was going to be dead. I did not want to die, but I was convinced I was going to. Now! At that moment, the implications of what this meant were rather vague to me. Like most urban, twenty-first-century Westerners, my experience of death was filtered through Hollywood where the streets were invariably bloody and violent, strewn with bodies either shot or crushed in car chases, and then miraculously vacuumed out of sight and out of mind. Like the unaccountable disappearance of dead birds which one never saw falling out of the sky. Funerals, if they were even a part of the narrative, always appeared antiseptic. The media in general offered us cleansed versions of "passing." We had strayed so far from "the farm," "the harvest," "the product of our labours," I thought, we wouldn't know a cow pie if we stepped in it.

The closest I had come to death was largely through "memorial services" or "celebrations of life." Some of those had been gut-wrenching, some tip-toe walks in the park. None had prepared me for my own encounter with death. We are a culture fond of euphemism. I suspect a good old-fashioned wake, pints hoisted, voices lifted in song, would have been a lot more satisfying. And real.

I remembered the wonderfully ironic poem by E.E. Cummings, "dying is fine) but Death":

> dying is fine) but Death
>
> ?o
> Baby
> i
>
> wouldn't like
>
> Death if Death
> were
> good:for

when(instead of stopping to think)you

begin to feel of it, dying
's miraculous
why?be

cause dying is

perfectly natural;perfectly
putting
it mildly lively(but

Death

is strictly
scientific
& artificial &

evil & legal

we thank thee
god
almighty for dying

(forgive us,o life!the sin of Death

I had taught this poem to my students for years. I had always thought its quirky playfulness pretty much self-explanatory, but in the waiting room the subtlety of the distinction between "dying" and "Death" took on an immediacy I had never had to confront in the classroom. How presumptuous I had been to expect eighteen- or nineteen-year-old students in a freshman English class to fathom such a complex metaphysical idea. Happily and rightly so, they were in the clutches of "living."

When my father was nearing the end of his life, the last fifteen years having been spent living with Parkinson's disease, I asked him one sunny, fall day while we were out driving if he was afraid of dying. I assumed that having lived with Parkinson's for so long, this was something that must have occupied his thoughts fairly regularly. I was curious about death, as I think we all are in our own way, although I don't recollect why the subject seemed so urgent at that moment. I think it was a question I had been asking myself for some time, but it was one nobody I knew wanted to discuss.

My father was in his early seventies at the time. He first looked at the dashboard, then out the window and then he turned and stared at me blankly, as if I were as thick as a post. He took a few deep breaths, sighed, and said nothing. I hadn't meant to be insensitive, and I don't know if he resented the question, but he never gave me an answer. His silence on the subject was not uncommon; it was more the rule than the exception. In spite of this moment of awkwardness, he was a gentle, good man, a conscientious objector during the Second World War who ended up as a draughtsman in a Boeing aircraft plant designing parts for B-52s. This irony was not lost on him.

By the time he died, dementia had claimed him and I doubt that his death mattered much to him. In fact, it might have been a relief.

My own response to the idea of dying had always been one of ambivalence. While I felt the chill of physical extinction, of no longer being able to do something as simple as fill my lungs with the smell of freshly mown grass on a summer morning, I took some measure of comfort from the teachings of the Buddhist master, Thich Nhat Hanh, in his book *No Death, No Fear.* His teachings guide us towards an understanding of death, but more importantly, encourage us to stop fearing life:

> Our greatest fear is that when we die we will become nothing. Many of us believe that our entire existence is only a life span beginning the moment we are born or conceived and ending

the moment we die. We believe that we are born from nothing and that when we die we become nothing. And so we are
filled with the fear of annihilation.

The Buddha has a very different understanding of our existence. It is the understanding that birth and death are notions.
They are not real. The fact that we think they are true makes a
powerful illusion that causes our suffering. The Buddha taught
that there is no birth, there is no death; there is no coming,
there is no going; there is no same, there is no different; there
is no permanent self, there is no annihilation. We only think
there is. When we understand that we cannot be destroyed,
we are liberated from fear. It is a great relief. We can enjoy life
and appreciate it in a new way. (4)

With these teachings in mind, I felt surprisingly tranquil for someone who was suddenly experiencing a premonition of his own end.

My body slumped back in my seat.

The couple next to me exited their phone booth and gaped at
me. I remember thinking, maybe they're worried that I'm infectious. What an odd thought to have.

Then I saw Pat running from one vacant desk to another. She
was becoming a blur.

I could hear her calling for help.

At that moment, I was almost flat out on my chair, slowly sliding
to the floor.

Then suddenly the room flooded with intense white light, the
sort of stylized light one expects to see in an avant-garde Italian or
French film.

Almost immediately I was surrounded by a number of very attentive, caring and skilled people who hoisted me with amazing ease
onto a stretcher — I'm not exactly an easy or light load to shift —
and whisked me into a treatment room where they inserted an IV
into my arm and attached me to several monitoring machines. I
could hear bleeps and beeps and hoped with all my might that they

were monitoring me. At the same time, everyone kept assuring me I was in good hands, a claim I didn't doubt then, and one I seldom had cause to doubt in the coming months.

My memories dim a bit at this stage. In an increasing haze, my new existence as a "stroke survivor" was about to begin in earnest.

People buzzed around me, all very efficiently. The choreography had all the precision and beauty of bees in a field of lavender. I love bees and admire what they do. Around me people flew, each with an appointed task. The performance was dazzling. They appeared to know what they were doing.

"What's happening to me?" I asked.

Was that really me speaking, I wondered? If it was my voice, it sounded a lot like an old 78 phonograph record spinning at 33⅓ rpm. The words rolled and bounced around the room like tumbleweed blown on a desert wind. They had no traction, no weight, no body. No meaning. And yet they seemed heavy and thick at the same time. Like toffee or treacle. Was this how dead people spoke or communicated?

"Don't you worry, Hon, you're going to be all right," one of the nurses reassured me. "We're going to look after you."

Bright light filled the room and I closed my eyes. I heard the whoosh and swish of movement, of cloth rubbing against flesh, and I heard whispered chatter, none of which quite made sense. Occasionally I heard something that sounded like metal against metal, sometimes followed by a needle inserted into my arm.

In a lab, somewhere in the hospital, someone was performing an analysis of my blood. Someone possessed the first clues to what was happening to me.

The next thing I knew my clothes were being removed. Shoes and socks first. I didn't have to lift a thing. My rear end and legs were raised, my pants came off. My torso sat up, my arms rose above my head and my shirt slipped off.

I remember blinking against the light and looking around the room for Pat. She stood off in a corner, watching. I could sense that she was comforted seeing me in able hands, but I also read fear in her eyes.

"Aren't you a lucky man," the nurse who appeared to be in charge said, "you've got five women undressing you."

I like to think I found this suggestion both stimulating and erotic, that my libido leapt into action, but regrettably nothing could have been further from my mind. I think it was slowly dawning on me that my movement was no longer voluntary. I couldn't be certain of this, but why else were five women undressing me?

Yet I laughed and agreed. This image froze happily in my mind, because it was the last fully conscious thought I was to have for two days.

I remember the lights dimming and Pat departing. I remember her kissing me lightly on the forehead and waving to me at the sliding glass door just before she pulled the curtain closed. I remember her face disappearing and a clock on the wall edging towards one in the morning.

I was alone.

Even the hushed sounds of a busy emergency ward had settled in for the rainy November night. Everything seemed subdued, as if a blanket had been pulled up and over a body laid to rest. The place had become a corpse. The atmosphere in my room was oppressive — smothered and muffled.

I had been on my own before but until that moment never truly alone, at least as far as I could remember. I wanted to weep. Deep down inside, deep down somewhere, a cord had been severed. Where exactly that place was, in the body or in the mind, I don't know. I was overcome by a heavy sense of loss. As I say, I wanted to weep, but the tears just wouldn't come. I lacked the strength, perhaps the will, to manage even that.

How to explain? Where are the words, the images? Everything was such a jumble then; and memory remains so confused. This all sounds so indulgent and melodramatic now. But at that moment, this is how I felt: empty, hollow, gutted.

Cut adrift.

It wasn't that I felt betrayed or abandoned. Quite the contrary. I definitely hadn't been. I knew I was loved. And yet, I felt as though I were trapped or lost at the heart of a maze. Bewildered, I couldn't see a way out. And I kept spiralling down, down to a place I knew I didn't want to go. It was so dark and crushing and lonely.

My experience that night is obviously why anti-depressants are one of the first medications prescribed for stroke victims.

Throughout that first night I have recollections of being shunted from my cell through the beige, brick and green hallways of the hospital and ushered into elevators, of being lifted and transferred onto the bed of a CAT scan machine. Back and forth I went through a fluorescent glare, never fully conscious of where I was going or what was being done to me. I assume I had been rather heavily sedated, undoubtedly a good thing I suspect, or I may have plummeted even further into that widening black hole that engulfed me. While I admit to being moody, I'm normally fairly upbeat, in an oddball sort of way, so this uncontrollable descent was frightening.

As best I could, I remember curling up, thinking my version of the prenatal position offered me the most reliable protection against free fall.

When Pat returned to the hospital in the morning, I was still in emergency. Although I don't recollect the precise time she walked into my room — Room 22, a master power number (Pat had always been fascinated with numerology, and 22 was a number that had probably brought me luck, she told me) — I remember being surprised that she had returned so early. The past twenty-four hours had folded so many events into such a short space of time. I was learning that time is pliable and multi-faceted in spite of the many ways we contrive to measure it accurately . . . to the nanosecond.

She told me the doctors had pretty much confirmed the original diagnosis — I had suffered a stroke. How severe it had been, no one knew. That was yet to be determined. And it would be at least another thirty-six hours before I would be told what I never, ever thought possible: that I might be paralyzed on one side of my body.

Paralyzed!

Not in my wildest dreams had I ever contemplated this outcome — debilitated, incapacitated, disabled, stunned, knocked out, anaesthetized, arrested, halted, addled, crippled, dazed, disarmed, frozen, deadened.

The words bounded from one corner of my brain to another, freewheeling, as if seeking an orbit that would make sense of this news.

How was it possible that no one knew?

In that windowless, white cubicle there were no distractions; silence was interrupted by the occasional beep that came from a monitor.

Soon I was to learn that not only could I not move, but when I went to form words, my tongue was unable to give them the shape of understanding. Words, treasured words, sounded like a cat being swung by the tail or the noises made by howler monkeys. My vocal cords seemed to be twisted. My words strangled. This punishment seemed doubly cruel.

Later on, this loss would come to mean, as far as I could see, a future held in abeyance, and a past at risk of being neglected.

Or forgotten.

All I wished to do at that moment was close my eyes and sleep.

TWO

The Room at the End of the Hall

Let me say from the outset that even though faced with chronic underfunding, hospital personnel and health professionals, at least throughout most of the First World, are incredibly dedicated and efficient; never has a population received such informed and, often, inspired care.

That said, for various reasons, some good, some bad, hospitals are not built for comfort. On the positive side, contemporary theory is that everything and anything should be done to hasten a patient's recovery and discharge. In the majority of cases, I'm all for that! Mind you, within the public system there are times when the squalor and congestion in hospital wards should shame us: beds in hallways, storage rooms and closets, bedding unchanged, patients unwashed. Sometimes the list gets embarrassingly long, especially for a society hoarding or squandering so much wealth. We know, though, that the faster a patient is forced to her or his feet, the quicker the healing process begins. In other words, the shorter the time a patient is dependent on the health system and returns to the healing powers of the familiar, of home and loved ones, the better. I think it would be fair to characterize this attitude with the motto: "Out of bed, on your feet, and out the door," with a subtext which should include, "and into the bosom of family or community."

Of course there are times when this theory doesn't make sense and is simply at odds with any acceptable definition of a caring and compassionate community. When people need extended care, the system needs to do better. Ushering a person out the door to the tune of some bureaucrat's beautifully orchestrated time study can create more angst than benefit and, in many instances, may be downright cruel. Clearly there are occasions that cry out for prolonged care and empathy, when the sharpened pencils of accountants are better tucked back behind the ear or shoved into the breast pocket, and we actually show as much concern for a fellow human being as we invariably show for a family pet. Some patients need constant care and attention, especially, for example, when they are in the grips of a life-ending illness, dementia or uncontrollable pain.

Or, as I was soon to learn, when they have had a brain attack — a more precise name for a stroke, "stroke" connoting a gentle or soothing action — and may not quite know who or what they are! Or, put another way, may suddenly feel they are not of this world.

As I lay in emergency, I was beginning to get the first inklings that this described me. The one thing I knew for certain was that I was losing something. I didn't know what or how, but something had gone amiss. We say, "He's lost his mind" or "He's out of his mind," but this usually means he's found "anger" or "become deranged" in some embarrassing way. For me, the confusion was overpowering and the loss profound. I wasn't finding or becoming anything. I was pretty sure I knew where I was, but not why I was there. Everything seemed so vague. So intangible. So mind-bogglingly alien, as if I was from another planet. Nothing made any sense, no matter how hard I struggled to slot a sight or sound or feeling into a compartment of my brain.

My term in emergency lasted less than twenty-four hours, yet what played in my scattered recollections felt like one of those illustrated tapestries from a school textbook that recorded several lifetimes. The one constant in my confused and clouded memory of that time was Pat. Seated on a chair pulled up to the edge of the bed, she floated in and out of view, mixed in with the sounds of sirens, of new patients being stretchered in, of the faint but urgent voices of doctors and nurses attending a new casualty, of whimpers from someone in pain, of pleas for help, of a baby crying, always a baby crying — all the general hubbub associated with a place dedicated to coping with chaos and misery.

Ironically, it's the sounds I remember, not the images. Every noise, whether water running from a tap, the swish of clothing, a code call over the PA system or a bedpan falling to the floor, startled me. When I did manage to open my eyes, everything dissolved into a collage or mishmash of light and blurred objects. Nothing in the visible world would hold still, would come into focus. Doubtless this had a lot to do with the medications on which my brain and body now depended.

Losing the visible is terribly disorienting. I can't imagine being blind. I realized as I was lying there that I take most of my cues — spatial, time, shape, colour, relationships (between objects as well as my connections to others), distance, absence — from what I see. What I see pretty much locates me in the world, is the primary way I know the world, and when I lost that connection, well, I became disconnected. Or unplugged. This sounds so simplistic, but that is what I was beginning to feel. Unplugged.

I remember craving sleep. From time to time, as I drifted to the surface of consciousness, I was of two minds. I desperately wanted to make contact with Pat, who watched over me like the Archangel Raphael. And I wanted to rest my head in her lap, although I wasn't quite sure how to accomplish that. Such a simple act eluded me. But then I also wanted to slide away, just slip off into what I can only describe as nowhere. I wanted to be anywhere but where I was. I struggled mightily with these two impulses.

Sleep, for which my brain seemed starved, generally won out.

Towards the middle of the afternoon of November 20th a woman came to Room 22 and said I had been assigned to a bed on the fourth floor of the main wing. She was not a nurse; she was one of a few people whose sole job was to wheel patients from one appointment to another throughout the vast network of byways that connect the various departments of the hospital. Someone later told me she was a porter, but in the fog that kept rolling onto the shores of my mind she and her mates became pilots who escorted me through the increasingly complex waters of confusion. And to all the tests!

I kept trying to make connections that simply did not link up.

On a couple of occasions the previous night, I had been transported to imaging and X-ray, past admittance and the coffee bar, where I had grabbed at the scent of the freshly roasted coffee that hung in the air. I needed something familiar to hold on to. I remember thinking at the time that escorting those facing an imminent operation or, more acutely, the ill and gravely ill must be unbelievably stressful, not unlike the role of an executioner's assistant. Just manoeuvring the length of a stretcher around corners and past those on a "Sunday stroll" required patience and skill. But carrying the extra burden of knowing this might be a person's final journey had to be nerve-racking if not emotionally numbing. Yet every one of these good souls I met, at least on my many expeditions through the hospital maze, was unflappable and cheerful; they often chatted away about the weather or offered encouragement like a football coach running up and down the sidelines during a match.

I came to love these forays into the unknown. The view from where I lay on my back as we careened around the twists and turns of the hospital corridors had an element of mystery and surprise. I had the sensation that I was floating, that I was being chauffeured about the heavens on a pillow of cloud.

In preparation for my move to the fourth floor, Pat packed my belongings in a plastic bag, and the porter, Pat and I became a little procession of pilgrims headed to the tower where serious medicine was practised. Once again I was on the move, all a part of the hurry-up-and-wait routine invariably at the heart of larger institutions.

Now I was about to enter a version of the hospital far too frequently reported on in the news: a terribly overcrowded, under-funded rabbit warren of hallways and small but functional rooms. As we rolled out of the elevator into the acute care ward, we passed the main nursing station and then wove our way between people shuffling along in night gowns and slippers, like sleepwalkers, pushing poles with various drip bags hanging from them; patients in wheelchairs navigating around nurses scrambling to respond to a buzzer or flashing light; therapists helping patients take that first step back to the promise of walking; cleaning staff trying to keep up with the latest mishap; and visitors, anxious to perform their duty and be on their way.

Who could blame them for their need to escape? Hospitals tend to overwhelm the senses, and, no matter how hard everyone tries, dampen the spirits. It's not the stink of decay or antiseptic that smothers our goodwill; nor is it hearing cries from patients in excruciating pain or seeing bodies lurching about like zombies in some terrible horror flick that kills our altruism. For the most part, hospitals are noisy and efficient, running on their own clock. What makes us skittish and tense is being witness to time in stasis. Before long, waiting over someone confined to a hospital bed can begin to seem too much like attending vigil over one's own future. A prelude. Who needs reminding of their own mortality? We become anxious to return to the world, to be a part of its ebb and flow.

As we glided along I glanced from side to side. From what I could see, the place was a madhouse. Mind you, everything was filtered through layers of gauze and I suspect my mind played with the tempo of things.

Slowly we made our way to a room at the end of the hallway, as far away as possible from the mayhem at nursing central.

"Aren't you a lucky man," the porter said, "you've been assigned to a double room. And the window bed, to boot!"

She appeared happy with this outcome, and I sensed I should be grateful for my good fortune.

"You'll only have to share the bathroom with one other person."

It wasn't at all clear to me why she considered this such a stroke of luck. I do recall thinking at the time that the phrase "stroke of luck" implied a terrible pun. And irony. What good was a semi-private bathroom to someone who was beginning to sense that he couldn't move because of his stroke, that he was now someone who might be dependent on others to assist him with the most basic of movements and bodily functions?

Over the past few hours, I had been wrestling with the idea that I might be paralyzed. What would I do if I were? When I wiggled my toes, though, I thought I could see them move under the sheets. But to be honest, I was simply too tired to know what to think.

A room with a view overlooking other rooftops, the cityscape and snow-capped Mount Benson in the distance was of little interest to me.

I hungered for two things: sleep and silence.

As soon as I had been transferred from the stretcher to the bed, a curtain was whipped around its track and I was partitioned off from the rest of the room. I didn't even catch a glimpse of my new roommate. I'm not sure we ever spoke, but it didn't matter. Within no time at all he was gone. I don't know to where, but for some reason I seem to think he was dashed away to intensive care. I had heard whispers, bits of conversation, as two nurses worked within inches of me behind the drawn curtain.

Conjecture, I was to learn, is one of the survival strategies of being a patient, perhaps because it's reassuring to think you're better off than someone else. Things could be worse!

A nurse who had assisted with my transfer to the bed introduced herself and explained that this room would probably be my home for the next three weeks. I remember staring at her as if she were speaking a foreign language. Mandarin or Latin or Swahili, take your pick, it didn't matter. She might as well have said forever, or eternity. Three weeks! Three weeks meant nothing to me. I let out a long sigh, not out of exasperation but from sheer exhaustion. Never had I felt so tired.

I wanted to swim out to sea and sink to the bottom where I imagined I would find peace and quiet.

The nurse was a hefty woman, tall, roundish, in her mid- to late-twenties, I guessed, and with kindly eyes. She was all business as she put everything in its place: my IV, the stand with drip bags containing nourishment, my chart, the sensory patches that sent my vitals to nursing central. It made me dizzy to listen to her movements and to watch her when I was able to keep my eyes open.

"If you need assistance just press this buzzer button, here on the pillow by your ear, and someone — probably me — will come running."

I don't know what kind of magician she figured I was. Not only couldn't I see the button, I couldn't reach it; and if I had been able to reach it I lacked the strength to press it.

Pat, who had spent the day with me, fussing over me, trying to console me, following my impromptu moves about the hospital, stood at the end of the bed, her shoulders hunched, with the weight of what was being said and happening to me pressing down on her. Everything had become so heavy. Like somebody had cranked up gravity. A feather could have knocked her over.

Although I had lost track of time, I knew it must be late in the afternoon as I watched the last, soft grey light, so typical of the West Coast at that time of the year, fade from the sky. Ah, I remember thinking, the window was of some use after all. As my mind rambled from thought to thought and drifted in and out of consciousness, I watched raindrops slide down the glass. Each followed its own path and then petered out. A window of disappearing rivers.

I could see Pat was anxious to get home. She already faced a rainy commute in rush hour.

"Nicole will be here tomorrow around noon. She called back to confirm she'll catch the 10:30 ferry."

I nodded. She was referring to our daughter, an archaeologist, living in Vancouver. Nicole's image came quickly to mind, although what I conjured up was a sketchy portrait at best: she had long brown hair, usually tousled; green, tidal-pool eyes; and she was tall and slim. Beautiful to my fatherly eyes, although she never dressed that beauty. She was too busy on "digs" and exploring clam gardens. I remembered that.

But "called back" made no sense.

Pat quickly detected my confusion. "You talked to her earlier today. When I called to tell her about the stroke."

Had I?

How could I forget that?

What had we talked about? My daughter, who I love dearly: what had we talked about? I drew a blank. It was not like me to forget any of our communications. I always teased her with some sort of silliness, but now nothing came to mind. Maybe I had pointed out again my dismay at the endless cycle of colds our granddaughter brought home from her contact with other toddlers at school. I felt little Flora was sickly far too often. Her playschool, one of the best in the city, could be a germ factory. But weren't they all like that? I could be really annoying on the topic. Why, I wondered, was I like that?

Or maybe I had asked about Iain, my daughter's partner, who was completing work on his PhD thesis. He was writing on some esoteric aspect of the herring fishery, which had been decimated over the last fifty years, a topic that should have been of concern to anyone interested in the resilience of salmon runs up and down the Pacific Northwest Coast and the health of the planet in general. He was from San Francisco and was a good father, I remembered that. He was researching the fish's role in the lives of First Nations peoples over the past ten thousand years of coastal history. I knew this was interesting and important work, but I was anxious for him to complete his research. Why was I trying to rush him? I could be relentless on the subject.

Why did I harp on things that were none of my business?

Were these the subjects we discussed? How would I know? I had only a vague recollection that we had even talked. And that only because of Pat's prompting.

What did her voice sound like? Had she mentioned anything important that I needed to remember? What was it? Why was I having so much difficulty remembering?

Questions flashed like Christmas lights. Red then green then red, and so on. Where was the amber? No, no, that was another kind of light.

I wanted to sleep.

"She'll drop Flora off at playschool and go directly to the ferry."

The information I was receiving seemed endless, seemed far too much to digest and remember. I yearned to close my eyes, but as long as Pat remained I felt obligated to stay awake. She was torn, I could tell, between going and not going. We were in a game of tug-of-war. I think she feared she would be abandoning me, that I would see her departure as a need, on her part, to escape.

Finally I said, "Go. Please. Go, I need to sleep."

She kissed me, lingered over me, looking into my eyes, searching for a sign that would tell her that it was okay to leave, and then she slid along the length of the bed and disappeared beyond the curtain. I waited. A few seconds later the corner of the curtain parted slightly and she peered in on me. My head lolled to one side and I watched her through my eyelashes. I didn't want her to know I still hovered on the edge of sleep. That I expected her to return. That I understood her mothering instinct.

She looked so, so tired.

And then she was gone.

Sometime in the early evening I was awakened by a commotion in the other half of the room. A new tenant was being moved in behind the curtain. Someone with whom to share the bathroom. What was this pretense to privacy?

His arrival came with all the fanfare accorded to a celebrity. He seemed to be setting up court and the chatter that surrounded him sounded like the fuss made by birds building a new nest. In spite of my overpowering desire for sleep, I struggled to focus. Why was he receiving all this attention? Who was he?

The one thing I knew for certain, he was loud.

"What am I doing on the fourth floor?" he asked.

"This was the only available room," a nurse answered.

"Usually they send me to the sixth! No insult intended, but they know me on the sixth. I know them. This doesn't make any sense."

"We'll do our best to get to know you Mr. . ."

I didn't catch his name, nor did I much care. I just wished he would dial it down.

"On the sixth, they know when and how to drain me."

"I'm sure we'll manage. You need to get some rest. And the gentleman next to you needs sleep. Plenty of sleep."

I heard her pull back the curtain to check on me and I waited to hear what he would make of this piece of information. There was a brief pause, but it became immediately evident that I was the least of his concerns. I imagined him flicking the back of his hand in my direction as if batting away a no-see-um.

"On the sixth they know when I need water," he said. "Sometimes they bring me juice. In spite of what the doctor says."

His voice faded in and out. My head felt heavy against the pillow, and I realized I was unable to roll on my side. How was I going to sleep if I couldn't roll onto my right side? At that moment this seemed a huge dilemma, a challenge to my familiar routine. I always slept on my right side, facing away from Pat. My eyes closed and the two voices beyond the curtain spoke in counterpoint to my brain seeking sleep. But there was no music in this composition, only the clash of multiple forces creating a terrible cacophony in my head.

"But you're to limit your fluid intake, especially juices. Our instructions are very specific. Very emphatic. The doctor's underlined it on your chart."

He sighed.

"I get thirsty . . ."

"I understand that, but the doctor has strictly forbidden juices."

"And I need something to break up the monotony of water water water."

"I can't . . ."

"Just a little juice box every now and then. They did that for me on the sixth!"

I could envision his lips curl back in a pout. The man was shameless.

"Well, we'll see, but I . . ."

"Thank you. You have no idea what a relief a little sip of orange juice or apple juice can mean to the taste buds!"

The nurse started to reply, but I imagined he disarmed her with a "cheesy" but purposeful smile. I already disliked the man.

"And the sugar. I need the sugar to keep up my strength," he added.

I was to learn this was his way of working the system. It was simple. He played floor against floor, nurse against nurse, and pitted nurses against doctors. He had manipulation down to a science. But more importantly, he basked in the attention it brought him. In the course of the next couple of days I watched and listened in awe as he kept a full complement of nursing staff at his beck and call.

For the moment, I drifted back into a light sleep, although I was constantly aware of his fussing on the other side of the curtain. And just when I did feel a deep sleep was within reach, he would jerk me back into his world as if my brain were on a leash without the will and wherewithal to wander on its own. I wanted to be free, I wanted to float off into space and find a corner where I could curl up with my own thoughts. Or with a mind blanked of thought. The idea that somewhere there was a place as black as a raven's feather teased my imagination.

But he wouldn't let me go.

When a nurse dimmed the lights in the room, it was a matter of seconds before he turned them back on.

"How am I expected to read?" he said, at the same time turning up the volume on his radio. Trickles of sound leaked out from around his earphones.

I couldn't see if there was a nurse present to hear him or not, but by this time he had my attention.

"I'd prefer them off," I said. "Both of them, the lights and your damn radio."

"What's that? What did you say?"

I knew what I was trying to say, but what I heard coming out of my mouth was incomprehensible, wasn't even in a language that I understood. It certainly wasn't English. Everything was totally garbled, was a total muddle. I could have been a sheep bleating for all the sense I made.

There was a brief silence as he shifted in his bed.

"You, on the other side of the curtain, what is it you're trying to tell me?"

I didn't think I had the energy to repeat myself.

I was frustrated. My thoughts were treading water and it was all I could do to keep them afloat.

I tried again, this time enunciating each syllable, as if addressing the village idiot.

"I . . . need . . . sleep."

I wasn't sure if this effort was any clearer than my previous pathetic attempt to communicate, but he seemed to understand.

"Right. Got you. I'll turn the sound down, but I'm keeping on the lights on my side of the room."

What was it he didn't understand? He seemed to miss the point entirely. Deliberately so. We shared the room and consequently shared the light. By now it was close to midnight and our room was lit up like a used-car lot. The only thing missing was streamers. All I wanted was for darkness and sleep to envelop me.

"I gather from what you're struggling to say that you're not an insomniac?"

"No," I said. I had the distinct impression he was toying with me.

"Too bad," he said, "I am."

He chuckled and I didn't know whether to take what he said as a simple statement of fact or a threat.

I wondered what his insomnia had to do with anything. What I did realize then is that he had control of the situation and relished it.

I knew he couldn't see me, but somehow he had figured out that I was more disabled than he was. Insomnia and dreams are flip sides of the same coin. With insomnia you are stuck in the real world, facing a growing urgency that nothing is likely to change, knowing you are trapped inside an uncompromising reality, while in the world of dreams you can at least escape into an imaginary realm; you can flee to where all the variables of imagination exist beyond space and time but, and here's the catch, whether you're an insomniac or dreamer sleep can become a nightmare. Monsters and gremlins can invade space at either end of this continuum.

For me that is exactly what sleep became, a hellish dream. During two of the longest days of my life, when I was as defenceless as I've ever been, my "roommate" and I were to haunt the same nightmare.

I managed to close my eyes, but his presence was always there, on the edges of sleep, dream and the room. The rest of the space, a humungous cavern, he filled with a fear of whatever it was he was suffering from. There was no point in pretending to sleep in the hope that he would follow my example, because he could concentrate only on his own pain and do whatever it took to lessen that. As the night wore on, and I caught spells of real-time sleep, I began to realize that everything he did was a distraction. The lights, the music, the countless requests for water and juice all helped him to cope, kept him occupied. My weariness was not his concern.

He did not see his interruptions as malevolent or even irritating; they were part of a game to which he had the only rule book.

At regular intervals, a nurse would arrive to remove a vacuum bottle of fluid from near the floor at the foot of his bed. It was at a level where I could just see it dangling beneath the skirt of the curtain. He and the nurses continued to play a game of dueling lights. And every so often they had to ask him to turn down his music. Pop tunes from the eighties and nineties could be heard throughout the ward.

This battle continued throughout the night until first light broke through the window, a pale winter light, and the rest of the fourth floor buzzed into life. Then things on his side of the room went surprisingly quiet. He had actually fallen asleep. Perhaps it was the natural light that gave him peace. He had witnessed the rise of another day.

I realize now he may have had a legitimate reason to fear the dark.

THREE

A Bear of Very Little Brain

In spite of the pandemonium that surrounded me, when Pat arrived mid-morning of the next day, I had managed a few hours of interrupted sleep. My sense of what had been going on was that I had been repeatedly tugged out of sleep into some diabolical experiment, in which I was both subject and witness, or into an interrogation to which I had no answers. My brain was rapidly hatching ideas that made no sense. Questions, harmless questions, incomprehensible questions, were repeated over and over. By everyone, it seemed, who chanced on my room or who was instructed to check in on me. Why, I wondered, couldn't they post my responses in a convenient place for everyone to read? Most worrying was what would happen if I gave a contrary response? Would I fail the test, whatever that was?

Someone had arrived at the beginning of their twelve-hour shift, at about seven I think, to take my blood pressure, pulse and blood for a blood sugar test. This monitoring four times a day would be continued for several weeks. Later I was told that stabilizing blood pressure and blood sugars in diabetics is vital to averting further strokes. And I think I was made to sit up and swallow several pills. I'm sure one of them knocked me out for the next three hours.

I was being drugged, I knew that. But why this was being done was still unclear to me.

When I woke up again and saw Pat sitting beside me, I was torn between panic and a huge sense of relief. Panic because the stark reality of what was happening to me was finally beginning to sink in — otherwise why would she be keeping such a close eye on me — and relief because my most reliable connection to the outside world, to a world to which I no longer felt I belonged, was seated at my elbow.

She would protect me, I was certain of that.

"I've had a stroke," I said.

This was a question as much as it was a statement.

She looked at me as if, like Pooh, I were a bear of very little brain. After all, she had already told me several times I'd had a stroke. But some notions are difficult to grasp, let alone accept, when you are trapped at the heart of a maelstrom of confusing and conflicting images and ideas.

"Yes."

Her answer seemed too quick, too glib. I was still hopeful that what had happened to me might be something else, perhaps a severe case of vertigo.

"They're sure?" I asked.

She nodded, unconvincingly, at least as far as I was concerned.

"You're sure?" I continued. "I mean, they've given you the test results?"

She shook her head slowly and looked past me, as if she were consulting one of those incomprehensible passages she loved from the

I Ching, cryptic words that somehow cast light on otherwise un-fathomable problems. Why was she being so evasive; why was she struggling so hard to answer me?

"Well," she said, "not exactly. No, not really." She hesitated. "But they know."

How? How could they know? Without proof?

"Somebody, a doctor, will be by the room this afternoon to talk to you. To explain what's happened," she said.

She hesitated, mulling over what she wanted to say next. Pat was usually one of the most confident people I knew, but now I could see doubt spreading across her face, like oil over water. Sadness over tenacity.

Today her high Nordic cheekbones seemed a little less high, a little less prominent.

"That's all I've been told. They don't say much. Nothing showed up on the CT image but that's not uncommon. It's all so confusing. I wrote to Edwin and Mary, and your family, and a few others friends to tell them you've had a stroke."

November 20, 2012

Hi Edwin and Mary,

Just a short note to tell you that Ron has suffered a stroke and is in hospital. Hopefully he will be able to come home in 5 days or so. At the moment he is getting good care. Nicole is coming over tomorrow and will be staying over-night.

Hope the news is better on your side of the pond.

Love,
Pat

Not for the first time I noticed her glance out the window at the low grey sky. Mount Benson was socked in, and a constant drizzle blurred what remained of the view. Rooftops, balconies, aerials, chimney stacks, a few evergreens.

"Do you understand me?" I asked.

She hesitated, as if she stood on the edge of a lake after a winter freeze and was about to walk out onto thin ice. She looked scared.

"Sort of. With a little effort I can make out what you're saying. It's difficult, though. Your speech is, well, a little impaired."

My speech was a little impaired! What exactly did she mean by that? Was that, as they say, like being a little pregnant? I had to admit, my tongue felt as thick as a pig's bladder and my mouth might as well have been filled with pebbles. Otherwise, what I was saying should have been perfectly clear. I had no trouble understanding what it was I was trying to say. Yet, as I listened, I could hear every word shoot out of my mouth like it had been fired with a rubber band. Syllables expanded and snapped in the oddest ways and seemed to fly off in every direction.

I paused and tried to organize my thoughts.

I wanted her to relax. I had to find a way to ease her mind.

Slowly, methodically, like an elephant walking, I said:

"I'm go-ing on a speak-ing tour with Step-hen Haw-king."

Pat laughed, her laughter a bit muted, but laughter all the same.

Then deliberately: "They're–going–to–confer–a–Doctor–of– Physics–on–me. It–has–something–to–do–with–our–respective– speech–patterns. Hawking–and–I–are–going–to–explain–the–ori- gins–of–the–cosmos. We'll–both–speak–like–this, with–no–inter- preter. It's–been–confirmed. It's–the–opportunity–of–a–lifetime."

For the first time since this whole business had started, she actually appeared composed. What a relief, for both of us. Her entire body settled, like a bag of feathers, as she let out a deep, deep breath. I'm not sure she understood everything I said; in fact, I'm pretty certain she didn't, but she caught the gist of it. I remember thinking that perhaps my difficulty speaking could serve as another defini- tion for tongue-tied. She told me later that this comment was when she first realized that I, the person she knew and loved, was still in there — she pointed at my head — and that my cognitive powers hadn't been damaged. She was certain then, and only then, that at least my mind, me, and my questionable sense of humour had survived.

But to be honest, the last few, long, long hours felt like I had been taken on a personal tour of a Hawking black hole. An emotional black hole as much as anything else.

With Pat nestled in beside me, I slept. Her presence provided me with a familiarity and protection I desperately needed. The constant hustle and bustle on the hospital ward was anything but restful. All that activity had purpose, constructive and positive, but it was not conducive to rest, which is the one thing a stroke survivor needs. Rest, and plenty of it.

With a stroke, the brain has taken a huge hit, a part of it killed. Destroyed. Erased. Snuffed out. Gone. Rubbed out.

You have lost a part of who you are.

Fatigue takes over.

Put simply, stroke is the wrong word. Attack, as in heart attack, would be more accurate. Attacked. Or ambushed. Your brain has been ambushed and you have suffered a brain attack. It is an attack every bit as serious as a heart attack. Perhaps more so.

Since having my stroke, I have learned that most people know what a heart attack is, or at least know that it is a serious, life-threatening business, but the word "stroke" is vague, is heart attack's lesser cousin. Because stroke is coupled with heart, it is viewed as cause for concern but less so. As I have said, stroke sounds soft, almost soothing. And without the word "brain" included as the part of the anatomy affected, it sounds like something external, like a light massage, perhaps. Like being petted. There is nothing in the word to alert you to the devastation it can wreak on every aspect of your being.

Most people, I concluded, don't know what a stroke is.

■

Weeks later, at the end of a day in therapy, when I was making some progress, I noticed a woman who had been admitted to the rehab unit around the same time as I was, sitting on one of the blue-matted exercise benches. The gym had emptied and was quiet, the way a museum can get near closing. Occasionally a voice could be heard shouting from one of the back offices where the therapists gathered. The woman's head was downcast and her posture was one of total defeat. Before I had my stroke I probably would have turned away, quietly, and left the room. I would have excused what I was witnessing as none of my business.

It's so easy to turn away.

She was slumped over as if she wanted to sink through the floor. I sat down beside her and rested my elbows on my knees. This was difficult because my right arm still wouldn't bend the way it was supposed to and still caused me considerable pain. It had the shape of a boomerang or chicken wing.

For over a minute we just sat there, staring at our feet, waiting, waiting as you do for the tide to come in or for the sun to set, waiting for the right moment to speak. Everything about the way she held herself worried me. You develop an unspoken bond with other stroke survivors that's impossible to explain. Perhaps soldiers on the front line in the Great Wars developed a similar intuitive sense and understanding with each other. How could they not under such terrible conditions? Rat-infested, muddy trenches. The open beaches of Normandy. Then I noticed tears running down her cheeks.

She was pale and her face was carved into the sort of chunks you sometimes see in a Francis Bacon or Picasso portrait. She had a modest beauty, one I suspect she had been unaware of or unconcerned about throughout her life. In the way that some people can be two things at once, she had an inner strength and outer timidity. Not a comfortable alliance at times, especially when raising children. She had two sons and a husband who visited her daily. She was one of the lucky ones. Doted on, from what I could tell, with great affection. And yet her once-striking face looked tortured and bruised from the inside out, her skin wrinkled and exhausted. Smoking hadn't helped.

"You okay?" I asked.

A foolish question, but I knew I needed to get her to talk.

"Yes."

She gave me a quick glance.

"No."

Now she studied me. Her grey eyes looked hollowed out and seemed to have sunk back into her skull over the past few weeks. Stroke survivors often take on a vacant look, as if they are absent from their own bodies.

"You're doing so well," she said. "I've been watching you."

She tried to smile, but the effort it took was too great, and her lips collapsed back into a grim line.

I had to admit, my recovery was going well. By that time I had begun to walk with the aid of a walker. I had pretty much abandoned my wheelchair and had started climbing stairs. I was pleased with my progress and pleased that someone else had noticed, but I never felt satisfied. In spite of my little successes, recovery was still a struggle.

"It's so difficult," she said. "I can't do what you do and we've been in here about the same length of time."

After a day's therapy, we'd often offered each other encouraging comments and occasionally exchanged bits of personal history as we wheeled back to the rehab unit. We didn't say much because we were generally too tired to socialize but she had said enough to convince me she was one of the survivors. She was going to make it over the wall. And out, back to a semblance of her old self.

"It's impossible for you to see how you're doing. You can't see yourself," I insisted. "You have to be convinced that you're making progress. Then you will," I said.

I understood this despair. I had gone through this conversation with myself many times. Only other stroke survivors knew what you were going through, but there just wasn't a vocabulary adequate to describe the ebb and flow of emotions. Manic moments were followed by overwhelming periods of doubt. You could slip below the surface, out of sight, so easily. Having a stroke was a nasty business.

"I've tried so hard. I do everything they ask of me. But I still need the wheelchair."

"Every stroke is different," I said, repeating the one tired answer that remained a constant in stroke dialogues, the one response which she didn't want to hear from me, not from someone who was actually living inside a stroke. What we shared deserved more than a platitude, more than a true-but-tired cliché.

I didn't know what else to say.

"It takes time," I said, fumbling over my words, perhaps taking the easy way out, "so much time, for all of us. You just can't give up."

As a stroke survivor you're constantly looking for positive reinforcement, not only from what you're achieving in therapy but from the determination of others. Everyone around you plays a role in your recovery.

"Before the stroke I had two heart attacks," she said. "Compared to this they were a piece of cake."

Then a sad look seeped back into her eyes.

"I thought it would be the same. But after both heart attacks I was back on my feet within a month or two. Not with this, though. I can't see a way out."

As if sensing danger, she visibly recoiled. Like a snail, withdrawing into its shell. She gave me her hand which was cold and bony. Then I felt her body shiver and stiffen, her lungs fill, her eyes stare resolutely into mine, and it was then that I knew that, despite her apparent despair, she would never give up. She was one of those people who in the face of terror find the strength to be brave.

"I just have to accept the fact that I'll never be the same. I'll never be the same person I was," she said. "Part of me has died."

She paused to try to take in fully what it was she had just admitted to herself.

"And I must remind myself that I can't do what you do," she added. "As you say, we're all different. Our brains are different."

Norman Doidge, in his brilliant book *The Brain That Changes Itself*, remarks: "In all of medicine, few conditions are as terrifying as a stroke when a part of our brain dies." (162)

Here's the problem: How do you tell other people, especially those closest to you, that the person they're conversing with post-stroke is not the same person they used to know? How do you tell them that it's not just a heartbeat you've missed? And how do you convince family and friends that a little piece of who you were has died, has vamoosed, and that you, yourself, are not sure of what's left of you? And, furthermore, that even you don't know what to expect of the new you. How do you explain this "little death" you've suffered without them thinking you've taken a short journey to La-La Land? You're not brain-dead, but your brain has been altered. As a stroke survivor all you can tell people is that you are as mystified by the experience as they are.

With time I began to realize that no one knows what a stroke is, at least not in any definitive way. A lot of guesswork is still involved, most of it based on solid if limited science. For the stroke survivor this may be the most challenging and eye-opening realization. I'm grateful to all the people who practise their branch of medicine on my behalf, but quickly I began to appreciate that, at best, the people advising me had a clinical understanding of what had occurred to me during my stroke. They could see evidence for their conclusions on an MRI or CT scan or in my behaviour, but what my brain would do in response to my stroke was a mystery, was largely uncharted. Largely unknown. In short, the brain is complex and relatively unmapped; it is the new *terra incognita*, capable, as Doidge shows us, of amazing transformations and equally staggering healing. As he points out, the work of researchers such as Michael Merzenich, Barbara Arrowsmith Young, Paul Bach-y-Rita, Edward Taub and many other pioneers working on brain plasticity and mapping the brain is nothing short of miraculous. What they've charted so far and are in the process of discovering is inspirational. Therein lies the future and the greatest hope for stroke survivors: the science of neuro-plasticity. With their help, with constructive guidance, I can see a future where stroke survivors will be able to heal themselves.

Even so, as a stroke survivor who is trying to recover from the "shell-shock" of a "brain attack," the one thing you do know with certainty is that you have not been stroked.

In the initial hours and days following my stroke, I wasn't quite sure what to make of people. Most words and actions made me feel uncomfortable. Almost everyone appeared to examine me as if I were an exhibit, as if I were disabled. Which, of course, I was. I had become overly self-conscious. Habits I had previously neglected to notice in those around me suddenly became visible. A way of standing; a way of pursing their lips as if preparing to whistle; a way of raising an eyebrow as if in reproach; a way of nodding their head as if saying, yes, yes, but . . . ; a tone of voice that sounded like a crow scolding or laughter that sounded like the tinkling of fine crystal. I noticed that sometimes what I had previously accepted as second nature now became either irritating or confusing. People could no longer hide from me. Secrets had been decoded. At the same time, I couldn't hide from them. My emotions were raw. In the coming weeks I noticed I wanted to weep when I saw a television commercial for starving children in Africa. Or when the news recorded another suicide caused by bullying. What had been distant or merely familiar in the past now began to live inside my skin. Perhaps for this reason, those closest to me became even more treasured. They had come to live in me in a way I didn't quite understand — their presence like discovering a pearl in an oyster.

I was looking forward to seeing Nicole and Owen. Pat had told me Owen, our son, had received permission to take time off from his work — he is with the police — and would be arriving in a few days. On the one hand, I was nervous, because I wanted them to understand what was happening to me, even though I didn't understand what was going on myself; on the other hand, I didn't want to scare them. The one thing I knew for certain, though, was that news of their imminent arrival brought me great comfort. The words "family" and "friends" took on an entirely new meaning.

FOUR

My Travels Begin

First I heard her voice exchange pleasantries with my roommate and then I looked up to see her face peek around the corner of the curtain. She was checking to see if she had the right room. She glanced quickly back and forth between her mother and me and then stepped towards us, her arms held out to her mother, an expression of concern on her face. Usually she greeted us with a confident smile, but today I could sense unease.

Although I wanted to leap out of bed and embrace her, hug her with all my might, all I could do was lie there like a beached whale. Once again I wanted to weep. It's unsettling to have your children see you so vulnerable. I had always presumed my daughter saw me as a figure of strength, as someone who would protect her, forever; as presumptuous as this must sound, I had never imagined our roles reversed. Now I was alarmed by the worry I read on her face. And by the role reversal. *She* was here to care for *me*. For a moment I felt desperate. Almost ashamed. Why I felt that way, I couldn't tell you. As silly as this sounds — it wasn't ego — I think perhaps it was more a sense of having let her down. Of disappointing her.

From the time she was a toddler and would stand rigid in a harness at the front of her baby buggy, leaning forward like the figurehead on the prow of a ship, Nicole combined an aura of serenity with quiet exuberance. And she always seemed able to temper this combination with a layer of good old-fashioned thoughtfulness. As we strolled along the edge of the road, facing traffic, in the seaside village in which we lived, she would greet other pedestrians and cars with a wave and a hearty "hello," confident her greeting would be returned with the same enthusiasm and joy. Usually it was. Now she was here to share her boundless optimism and to give me encouragement wrapped up in a couple of simple messages: "You're going to get better" and "We all love you."

I can't over-emphasize the importance of this kind of support to the recovery of the stroke survivor. To adapt an old Benjamin Franklin axiom, "An ounce of love is worth a pound of cure." A little hope and lots of love constitute a good part of what's needed in the stroke-healing formula.

Nicole inched along the side of the bed, leaned over and kissed me.

"Oh, Dad," she said, "I'm so sorry."

"Me too," I said.

My voice still sounded like I was chewing on a mouthful of rubber bands.

"Owen and Jen send their love, too," she said. "And Iain and Flora."

"I know," I said. "It's so good to see you."

Although I had only recently climbed somewhat groggily out of my first sound sleep in two days, a blissful sleep which had probably lasted no longer than a couple of hours at best, and while I was thrilled to see her, I remember the precise time of Nicole's arrival on the fourth floor because I was also famished. I hadn't eaten for two days. It was just past noon and it appeared they had forgotten me again. I had been wakened when the kitchen staff delivered a meal to my roommate. For the umpteenth time he had demanded juice. Everything seemed to stop with him, literally. And the smell of the broth lingered everywhere, as if it were being pumped through the air exchanger. I wondered why I wasn't a part of the rotation. I asked Nicole if she would mind fetching the nurse, the young one who had been so helpful since my arrival on the ward. I wanted to know why they appeared to be starving me.

Meanwhile, I turned to Pat, who looked as if she were at the breaking point in a marathon, when cramps set in and you just can't seem to get enough fluid into your body, and you can't see the end, the finish line. Immediately I recalled the one other time I had felt this hungry. While I think hunger has a way of etching itself into one's memory, the effects of the stroke kept dredging up random events from my past that I thought I had long ago consigned to the dustbin.

"Have I ever told you about that time in Paris when I passed out from hunger in the American Express office?"

I couldn't get over the sound of my own voice, the way I was mangling words as they stumbled off my tongue. And now my jaw felt unhinged, as if it might float away from my face.

"Yes," she said, "several times."

"Then I won't tell you again." I tried to say, "I certainly don't want to repeat myself. You might think I've lost my mind."

She sighed, put on her reading glasses and removed a book from her purse. I knew I could be exasperating, but where was the joy in being predictable?

"Cross-word puz-zles?" I asked, breaking up the syllables.

"No, Sudoku."

"Good brain ex-er-cise," I said.

The last time I had been as hungry as I now felt was during a trip a friend and I had made to Spain, Gibraltar and Morocco.

While Pat and I waited for Nicole to return with the nurse, I closed my eyes and searched through a reel of images that started in January 1965.

I was amazed by how much I remembered, in particular some of the details.

Just after New Year's, my friend, Jim, and I had left London and taken up residence in a cheap Paris hotel, somewhere in the student quarter. Overnight it turned cold and we woke up to find the city coated in a thin layer of frost. Under a blanket of white, the "City of Light" was magical but bone-numbing chilly. Ice had already formed in the bathroom sink.

Immediately we decided to head south to warmer temperatures. We figured the farther south we went the better, so we selected Malaga as our destination. We both had limited funds and we had heard from several contacts in London that Spain, even the Costa del Sol, was inexpensive.

On the morning of our departure we hitchhiked for well over two hours and yet we still seemed to be in the centre of the city. Each short ride felt like walking on a treadmill. Buildings were starting to take on a disturbing familiarity. Finally a blue and white police car pulled off to the side of the road in front of where we stood with our thumbs stuck in the air, both of us somewhat dejected by the whole experience. One officer got out of the car, opened the rear door and motioned for us to get in. From the smile on his face we hoped we weren't being arrested.

My French was pitiful, but Jim understood enough of what we were being told to realize we had spent the past couple of hours circling Paris on the ring road. They had seen us make one complete revolution. And apart from being puzzled by our behaviour, hitchhiking on the ring road was illegal! When we explained what we had been trying to do, they exchanged glances, all the time wondering if they should laugh at us or pity us, and then they escorted us to a road that actually led out of the city. To our surprise, they waved down a tanker truck and told the driver our story. He gestured for us to climb up and take a seat in the cab. He was headed down the Loire Valley, eventually all the way to Bordeaux.

What a break! This took a giant bite out of France. We thanked the two policemen, they wished us a safe journey, and we were on our way. I don't remember much of that long trip, although I do recall thinking this was rural France at its best. I remember vineyards and orchards rising away from the river like stick men, and neat fallow fields that I was later told were probably planted in the summer months with artichokes and asparagus.

We rolled through Orléans, Joan of Arc's town, and Tours, the driver as our guide, past one exquisite medieval château after another. This was a place of fairy tales, the true heart of France.

At one point the driver stopped to take a piss. He just pulled off to the side of the road and took care of business. Feeling a *sentiment de liberté* we joined him. He then unlocked a small door at the side of the cab and removed a bottle of wine. For half an hour we lounged at this lay-by, each of us taking a turn sipping directly from the bottle, and then he made a grand, sweeping gesture with his hand, indicating that this was his cargo. To our surprise, we had hitched a ride aboard a tanker truck filled with the same delicious wine we had just shared. For a moment we imagined ourselves pirates or hijackers and wondered aloud if it would be possible to make a getaway across the French–Spanish border with a truckload of liquid loot? What a way to arrive in the south of Spain. We laughed at this crazy but tempting idea and our new friend laughed along with us.

To this day I have no idea whether or not he understood what we were saying, but I suspect not and hope not, because he was filled with what I think the French mean when they use the phrase *joie de vivre*. Throughout the trip he belly-laughed from one moment to the next. He was a big jowly man, and when something struck him as funny, everything about him wrinkled into a smile, turned into a thousand crow's feet. Life had been hard — driving a big rig day in and day out had put a strain on his body — but he seemed satisfied to be happy. In the small hours of the morning, he dropped us off in the centre of Bordeaux, embraced us and, I assume, headed home.

This was an adventure. For the first time in our lives, Jim and I were living outside a routine, outside strict rules of conduct. Both of us had managed to catch a catnap on the drive south, albeit with one eye open. Now we needed a couple of hours of solid rest. Jim started pulling on the door handles of parked cars until he found one that was unlocked. Then we tumbled into the front and back seats and dozed until we heard the first sounds of a city waking.

Apart from the two apples we had "liberated" from a fruit vendor as we made our way to the ring road earlier that previous morning, and the wine we'd downed in the Loire Valley, neither of us had eaten all day. Now as we walked south, heading towards the outskirts of Bordeaux, following the route the tanker driver had sketched in the dust on the hood of his truck, we passed a bakery with baskets of baguettes in the doorway. A couple of steps past the freshly baked bread, we looked at each other, did a quick about-face and casually sauntered back past the entrance. There was no one in sight in the shop, everyone was out back attending to the baking, and the streets at that hour were empty. Hunger overrode guilt and we each nicked an oven-fresh loaf of crusty bread and set off at a brisk pace, behaving every bit like the two petty drifters we'd just become. I'm more inclined now to think we looked like a couple of giddy jackasses, but that's hindsight.

A few hours later we had managed to hitch several short rides past Bayonne to the turn-off to Biarritz. Natural light was disappearing quickly from the sky. I remember standing at the intersection between the main road and the exit, under the yellow glow of streetlights that had just come on, thinking how odd and quiet everything had suddenly become. I looked in three directions — there wasn't a car to be seen. Where was everyone? It was as if someone had decreed an end to the day and a clapperboard had sounded to terminate the action. It was absolutely still.

We had a choice, to head into Biarritz for the night or carry on into Spain.

Somewhat frustrated but determined, we began walking the eighteen kilometres to the border.

What surprised me, as I lay there in my hospital bed, was that I seemed to be able to recount these facts and details of fifty years ago without much reflection, with as much ease as rolling over and saying to Pat, I didn't get much sleep last night.

I opened my eyes just a slit. No Nicole, no nurse and still the hunger. Out of the corner of my eye I saw Pat working on her Sudoku. I could see that she was engrossed and, to my relief, distracted. I was only now beginning to fathom how demanding the life of a caregiver was likely going to be.

And then I returned to the south of France.

The word frontier suited perfectly this stretch of road. I couldn't remember ever having felt quite so solitary, not even in the northern, mountainous backwoods of British Columbia, in amongst the tall timber, rock and thick undergrowth. No, this road felt like it might actually disappear off the edge of the world. The January winds blowing in off the Bay of Biscay were bitterly cold; gulls were huddled white specks in the barren fields. Two things became apparent: south might not mean warmer, and we didn't have enough clothing to spend extended periods outdoors. I reached into my pack and pulled out another sweater. By this time, all remnants of daylight had vanished. Darkness wrapped around us like an icy cloak. I remember wondering how far we had walked, and thinking, what a dismal place.

And then, as if in answer to a less-than-hopeful prayer, a car came bouncing around a bend in the narrow road, a Citroën CV2, its headlights targeting first the pavement, then the hedges, trees and sky. It was the smallest Citroën model made, a light grey, and looked as if the suspension had been added as an afterthought — I imagined four coiled springs at each corner. It lurched past us, and kept going for several hundred metres before the brake lights suddenly lit up and the car came to a stop.

Half walking, half running, we closed in on the car. We didn't

want to appear too anxious in case the driver had stopped for another reason or might suddenly have second thoughts. When we
got close enough we could see him through the rear window turned
in his seat and beckoning us on with a quick flapping of his hand, as
if he were fanning himself. When we got to the open passenger
window, he smiled and said something to us in Spanish and kept
gesturing with his hands towards the seats, all of which we took to
mean, "hop in." Which we did, with a little effort.

Memory is a wonderful part of the brain's function, but when it
comes to precision sometimes it seems a bit of a blunt instrument;
on other occasions, with a little twirl of an inner wheel, it becomes
a tool of fanciful invention. While I remembered the make of the
car exactly, other details now slipped behind a fog bank. Facts took
on an aura of endless and exaggerated possibility.

Before we were picked up, we must have walked a fair distance
through the darkness along that lonely, twisting road, because within no time at all we were at the border. Ten minutes, at the most. I
was folded and tucked into the back seat like a hanky in a breast
pocket, my head rubbing against the canvas top, although in a CV2
no one really gets to stretch out.

We explained that we were Canadians — our driver spoke fluent
French — news which set him chatting away as if we were long-
lost relatives or neighbours. With him at the wheel, crossing the
border under glaring lights became a simple formality. Guards on
both sides knew him on a first-name basis, so while they exchanged
greetings and he told them who we were — what he could have
said about us, I have no idea — all that remained was for someone
from each country to stamp our passports. *Voilà*, we had been adopted. Everyone was quite friendly, some were outright jolly. We
had expected difficulties crossing the border. We were convinced
we would be hassled — two young males with longish, unkempt
hair, unshaven, carrying backpacks and sleeping bags spelled potential trouble. Instead, we were ushered on our way as if we had

arrived by invitation. Even a pair of the notorious Guardia Civil standing nearby in their three-cornered hats, holding what looked like submachine guns at the ready, paid us little attention. Entry into Franco's Spain couldn't have been easier.

Soon we were bounding down the road to San Sebastián, our new friend telling us in a flurry of French about this city, his home, that he loved and wanted to show off to us. His pride and confidence encouraged him to press the gas pedal to the floor. This was where he had been born, and his passion for the place radiated from him, outweighed any sense of caution he had as we sped towards the centre of this small but beautiful city clustered on the southeastern edge of the Cantabrian Sea.

Once parked, he led us to the harbour and onto an expansive promenade that ran for miles adjacent to the crescent-shaped beach. A northwesterly wind against which you could spread your arms and lean and remain standing funnelled in from the Atlantic. Wave after wave smashed against the stone wall that separated sea from land, each comber shooting fifteen to twenty feet into the air, casting an arc of spray and foam across the street. Up and down the walkway, groups of young people challenged the surge. Like surfers, they waited for a wave to crest, and then they ran from its lick that would have soaked them from head to toe had it caught them. I remember thinking, here we are, just arrived in Spain and already we're seeing a variation on a bullfight. Running with the waves was like running with the bulls, although I suspect fractionally less dangerous. What a spectacle; what a wild and playful night.

And then, another more sobering element was added to the composition — a long slanting rain mixed with sleet began to fall.

As the wind picked up speed and the temperature dropped to an uncomfortably damp and penetrating cold, our host suggested we seek shelter in a nearby tapas bar, one he frequented and knew well. He had friends he wanted to introduce us to. The moment we walked through the door, we could feel the warmth from bodies standing toe to toe, chin to chin, everyone with a glass of wine in hand, everyone involved in an intense conversation about family, politics, the price of land, a new building project, the cost of living, what folly so-and-so was up to — in short, the news of the day. All were men and at least half of them wore Basque berets, either black or navy blue.

Down the length of a long narrow room, dozens of cured legs of ham hung by heavy twine from the ceiling. A varnished wooden bar, ornate and polished to a high gloss, divided the space, one side for patrons, the other for the waiters who rushed about like a well-coordinated drill team and poured a local wine from what seemed like endless uncorked and ready bottles. Or was it barrels? Here memory plays one of its tricks. I do remember a handful of chefs, standing at a counter along the far wall, swiftly carving ham into thin slices which they then slapped into small buns. When one leg of ham had been eaten another was chopped from its mooring and readied for slicing.

Our host was a popular man. He knew everyone on both sides of the bar. When he walked through the crowd, there was no jostling. Space grew around him. Good-hearted and generous, when he shook hands with someone — to whom he would then introduce us, his new Canadian buddies — he did so with a sense of gratitude, with a grasp of the other's hand that confirmed his friendship. And after each introduction, as a token of that friendship, we were treated to another glass of wine. To our surprise and delight, each glass of wine was also served with a small, crunchy bun filled with one of the most deliciously exquisite slices of ham I had ever tasted. As hungry as we were, it soon became impossible to eat as fast as we drank. At first I carefully put spare rolls into my jacket pockets, something appetizing for the road in the morning. But as we progressed down the bar, I couldn't keep up with the production. I buttoned my coat, wrapped each new bun in a napkin and stuffed it inside my jacket. Given the way my girth was expanding, I would have enough ham-filled buns by the end of the evening to see me through to Madrid.

Eventually the wine took its toll. Both my bladder and my legs were giving out. Jim wasn't in much better shape. I needed a washroom and a breath of fresh air. As I stuck yet another bun into my jacket, I heard a voice.

"So, your daughter tells me you think we're starving you?"

This was not a voice from my memory. There had been no women in the bar.

"Now, why would we do that?"

The voice was soft and tender, diffused, covering me like a warm blanket.

My eyes blinked open and I saw Pat looking up from her book of puzzles. Then I saw the young nurse I liked so much leaning over me, smiling. Nicole stood at the end of the bed, her eyes, the same colour as mine, focused on me, waiting for my response. What seemed like a long silence followed. For some reason, I saw this as another test. Whatever I said, Nicole would parse and draw conclusions; she would know how well I was doing. She understood my humour and knew how evasive I could be.

"I don't know," I said. I tried to think of something wise to say, but my brain felt listless, as if it were dragging around a heavy sleigh of stones. "I don't know," I repeated, "but 'Please, ma'am, I want some more.'"

For a moment the nurse looked at me as though she was working out a riddle and then she said, "Of what?"

"Never mind," I said, pausing, wondering what it was I thought I had to prove. "Let's just say I'm hungry."

A little glint of light flickered in her eyes.

"Dickens, right? Very clever. I can see I'm going to have to be on my toes. I bet you thought you'd fooled me?"

Then she hummed a couple of bars of a song and flung out her hands: "I saw the musical."

She lifted my wrist and took my pulse.

"Never read the book, though."

I nodded. I was pleased. She *had* understood my reference to *Oliver Twist*, no matter what her source.

"Yes," I said, "you got it right. But I'm still hungry. Even a bowl of gruel would be nice."

"I know, I know." She patted me on the arm. "But we're not allowed to give you anything to eat. Not until the 'Swallow Lady' has been to see you."

I shifted beneath the covers as best I could and stared up at her, putting on a face I hoped might elicit a bit of sympathy. The sort of thing I had visualized my roommate doing for the past twenty-four hours. Non-stop. I could almost hear my voice dip and rise in a similar wave of pathos. Not unlike the sound old sea lions made when cast aside by the colony. What a chorus of brooding. Night after night during the winter months, I would lie in bed at home and listen to them moan and groan from an island about a mile off shore in front of our house. I loved that mournful sound. And I was saddened by it.

"The 'Swallow Lady' must decide," she said, jarring me back to the hospital room.

This was absurd. Now she was speaking in riddles. Or euphemisms. I shut my eyes. I had heard of a "Bag Lady," a "Lady of the Night," a "Pink Lady," "Lady Godiva," "The Lady of Shalott," "The Lady of the Lake," but I'd never heard of a "Swallow Lady." One part of me envisioned a small songbird, swift and acrobatic, that fed on the wing. I loved to watch them dip and dive as they picked off insects in an evening sky. The other image was a little more difficult to compose. I imagined a large figure covered in feathers, too large to fly. An emu, perhaps. She wore glasses and toted a clipboard under one wing and a pen under the other. Nothing made sense. Whoever this mysterious person was, she wielded a lot of power. Too much, I decided.

As I looked up, the nurse's smile broadened. It occurred to me that she might actually be enjoying my befuddlement, but instinctively I knew I was wrong. She was making me think, as exhausting as that continued to be. I began to realize she wanted to know if what I was saying was coherent. Or, perhaps, if I understood what she was saying.

"Swallow Lady," I said, "what in heaven's name is that? Or who?"

"The speech therapist," she said. "We need her authorization before you're allowed to ingest any food or liquids. She'll be by sometime today or tomorrow — she's very busy — to give you some tests to see if your swallow mechanism is working properly. We don't want you choking on your food."

"Of course I can swallow," I said. "Haven't I swallowed a bucket-load of pills in the last two days?"

"Yes, but that's different," she said.

"How?" I was growing weary. I could actually feel my mouth beginning to form into a pout. I was becoming a petulant brat. Worse than my roommate.

"Surely swallowing is swallowing," I said.

"Not always, sometimes it's not quite so automatic," she said. "This morning you experienced a fit of coughing after you took your pills. Remember?"

I did, but I failed to see the connection between my present hunger and the process of swallowing. Everything she said was beyond me.

More to the point, I wondered how it was she understood so easily what it was I was trying to say. My speech continued to be totally garbled. My teeth, tongue and lips were definitely at odds with each other. I could feel my mouth droop on the right side and the sag worsened with fatigue.

She later told me that listening to stroke patients required careful attention; you had to adjust your ears to nuances of sound. And understanding only came with plenty of practice. She had become accustomed to interpreting the slurs, changes in pitch and emphasis, dropped words, altered syntax and so on. Aphasia (a disorder caused by damage to the parts of the brain that control language) was particularly troubling because often patients knew what they wanted to say but couldn't find the words. Then she would have to enact what she felt the patient needed or wanted to say. Clearly this required a generous measure of empathy.

About one quarter of all stroke survivors suffer some form of language loss, but I suspect the percentage of people who experience a problem with swallowing (known as dysphagia) is much, much higher. A few studies suggest 65 percent. Based on my experience, I suspect everyone who has had a stroke may find, to a greater or lesser extent, difficulty swallowing. I don't think anyone has gathered conclusive statistics on the matter; testing a patient's ability to swallow has simply become a part of stroke protocol. And rightly so. The assumption is that if you've had a stroke your ability to swallow may have been compromised. Later I would come to appreciate how refined and remarkably coordinated the anatomy of swallowing is. But for the time being, as I lay there pondering my hunger, I was convinced I could eat a steak and wash it down with a fine glass of wine, on the spot; that is, if only I could cut it.

"So," the young nurse said, "I'm afraid you'll have to continue to take your nourishment from the IV. I know that's not what you want to hear — it doesn't fill the belly — but it's for the best."

My face must have expressed my doubt and disappointment.

"Really," she added.

I didn't quite know how to respond to this news.

"Okay?" she asked.

"Yes," I said, although clearly I wasn't pleased, but I knew I was pressing a point on which she was unlikely to budge and one that might get her into trouble. I lacked my roommate's persuasive powers.

"'Swallow Lady,'" I muttered, as the nurse disappeared beyond the curtain. "What's next?"

At that moment, I'm not sure that any additional information about the mythical "Swallow Lady" and her version of a medical panacea would have improved my mood or made the slightest differ-ence to my skepticism about what they were telling me. Put simply, I was hungry. And I couldn't see the harm in a bowl of soup, some-thing I was positively, unequivocally, emphatically certain I could swallow.

Nicole sat on the edge of the bed and studied me with a mixture of curiosity and concern, attentiveness and caution. She took my hand and squeezed it. Her response was understandable given my incomprehensible speech, my general confusion, my mumbling, my emotional fragility, my sudden mood swings and my stubbornness. It was as though I occupied both ends of a teeter-totter. Up and down I went, unsure of both. Up in the air I became giddy, like Humpty Dumpty sitting precariously on his wall, while down be-low I felt like a shadow-being existing outside of time and space. It was as though I had lost all dimensionality. I felt like an unusual artifact Nicole might unearth on an archaeological expedition, at the bottom of an excavation pit.

In what dim, dark past had I walked the earth? Could I be carbon dated? I had my doubts.

At that moment I was beginning to feel as though I no longer be-longed — to anything. This estrangement was not a case of my feel-ing sorry for myself. It was not solely an emotional issue, although the loss of emotional control played a large role in my increasing sense of alienation; it was equally a physical matter. A question of "being." Who was I and what was I? As absurd as it might sound, my mind began entertaining the idea that I was not a part of this world. Over the next few weeks this disengagement intensified, at least as far as I was concerned. And this is when my family — Pat, Nicole, Owen and eventually extended family, close friends and caregivers — tossed me a rope that would ultimately pull me back to the familiar.

In concert with all the medications, recovery strategies and ther-apies used in the treatment of stroke survivors, the most powerful elixir, the most effective antidote to the ravages of a stroke, what a friend has called the "carpet bombing" of the brain, is love. Love. Heavy doses of love and tenderness. And humour. It's that simple. Deep down, at the very bottom of the stroke void, there is a battle taking place, and without considerable emotional help and comfort the patient will lose that battle. Everyone — no matter what their association with stroke treatment, whether cleaners, nurses, kitchen staff, imaging technicians, doctors, therapists, family, friends — everyone who comes in contact with a stroke patient needs to be a part of the healing process. And the first step towards providing that essential support is visceral and unsentimental.

It's the giving of emotional commitment.

Pat, who was sitting quietly beside the bed, now doing a cryptic crossword puzzle — I always know when it's a cryptic puzzle she's doing by the way she chews the end of her pen or pencil and by the movement of her lips — stood up, looked out the window, and announced she was going for a walk. There was a break in the weather and she felt a need to stretch her legs. For the first time in days, sunlight streamed through a small crack in the clouds. A good brisk walk, she told us, a climb up the hill to the Chinese cemetery across the road from the hospital, would do her a world of good. Later she reported that she had also strolled through a beautiful, old grove of large arbutus trees next to the cemetery, all gnarly and twisted and growing out of what appeared to be solid granite. She marvelled at their adaptability and their peeling, rusty-coloured bark.

As she tied the belt on her coat, she said: "While I'm gone, your daughter will look after you." She bent over and kissed me. "Okay?"

I nodded and she brushed my cheek with her hand.

There was no question Pat needed to get away from the hospital . . . and me. She had kept a watchful eye over me without complaint, becoming a prisoner of her own resolute nature. I admired her strength and determination, her unwavering sense of hope, but everything has duration. Steadfast in her vigilance, she was like a robin guarding her nest against predatory crows. I had become one of those fragile, powder-blue eggs nestled in a bed of moss and twigs.

When Nicole arrived I saw Pat relax for the first time in days. Her shoulders settled, in the same way a cat's or dog's body settles into sleep in a pool of sunlight. She had someone else with whom to share her concern. Her love. In many respects, she was as much a captive of my damaged body and brain as I was. Only she didn't have to worry about or abide my roommate who I could now hear moving beyond the curtain. And she seemed to understand things that confused me. Without her the world would have become an unbearably bleak place, of that I was certain. I was happy she wanted to take this time for herself.

Besides, this would give me an opportunity to visit with Nicole.

What Nicole saw when she looked at me must have been scary. I was like an incomplete sketch of myself. Lines didn't meet up with each other, they didn't connect in the way they should have, giving the impression that my limbs were out of alignment, that everything about me was out of harmony. Unlike a photograph which, even though static, gives the illusion of being whole. Or, should I say, gives the illusion of a whole being.

Even my face was contorted, I could feel it, like I'd pulled on a rubber Halloween mask.

"What's that?" Nicole asked.

"What?"

"Your leg. You keep kicking or nudging me." She smiled. "Are you trying to give me a hint? Do you want me to leave?"

"No, no, of course not," I said. "Spasms. They're spasms. I can't help it. I can't stop them."

I was suddenly afraid she might leave. I struggled to find a way to let her know how much I wanted her to stay and how grateful I was that she had come to be with me. I wanted to reach up and straighten the tangle of fine hair that swept back behind her ear, but my right arm felt leaden.

Then she smiled again, the way I imagined she would smile at Flora, her three-year-old daughter. My granddaughter.

"Just teasing," she said. "Did you say spasms?"

I'd forgotten. My voice again.

I needed to speak more clearly.

"Yes. Like cramps," I said slowly, as if addressing someone new to the language. "They're involuntary. They're beginning to happen in my arm as well. And they hurt. They feel as though someone is jabbing me with a knife. Very unpleasant."

"Can't they do something?"

The tone of her voice had changed. I could hear and feel the strain. Her face, so young, had become a map of apprehension.

"I don't know. I think they've given me a muscle relaxant, but it's not working. Not all medications do what they're supposed to do. Or work for everyone."

Without warning, I started to cry, but not because of the pain. This surprising outburst came totally unbidden, as if something within me that protected me had suddenly broken down or a spring that held things together had sprung. Or recoiled. I simply lost control, and no matter how hard I tried I couldn't stop the tears.

I have no idea how long I wept.

I remember Nicole trying to console me. She wrapped her arms around me and held me, and I could feel a slight trembling from her chest.

Then as suddenly as the tears had come they stopped.

"How could I have been so stupid?" I said. "I should have taken better care of myself. If I'd taken better care of myself this wouldn't have happened. And you wouldn't have had to see me like this."

"Dad . . . ," she said.

I rambled on, repeating a chorus of regrets.

And Nicole did everything in her power to dissuade me of the blame I was determined to heap on myself.

What a way to behave. After all, she had dropped Flora off at daycare, and then she had driven through the congested heart of Vancouver, through Stanley Park, over the Lion's Gate Bridge, out to Horseshoe Bay where she had caught a two-hour ferry ride to Vancouver Island just to be with her father. With me. Three hours alone on the road, with time to think. I couldn't imagine what frightful images she must have conjured up as she tried to come to terms with all the permutations of what a stroke might mean. Paralysis, loss of memory, inability to speak or eat, problems with distance and depth perception, loss of vision, loss of balance and coordination, trouble breathing, on and on the list went. These were only a small number of the effects caused by trauma to the brain. One horror after another must have played itself out as she searched the Internet to understand what might be happening to me. Now I was being unfair with my litany of self-recriminations. At the time, I had no idea that this was typical behaviour for someone who has suffered a stroke. Nor did I realize that the spontaneous melancholy I had just experienced, often accompanied by an uncontrollable rush of tears, was something I would experience for months to come.

Chilled and perplexed, I closed my eyes and tried to curl up, although my body was having trouble obeying my wishes. Beyond the curtain that separated us, my roommate woke up briefly to demand a juice box. Already I was dreading spending another night with his insomnia.

Shortly after Pat returned from her walk, a young doctor, a physiatrist (a specialist who treats the patient as a whole through rehab medicine) appeared at the end of my bed. He was lean, had reddish-brown hair, and shuffled along in his sandals with the poise of someone who expected to be listened to and heeded. He looked like he could have walked off the set of a Hollywood soap. As he spoke, he bent the elbow of his right arm, held it with his opposite hand, and reached up to tap his chin with his index finger. Like Jack Benny had done years earlier, on black-and-white TV, during his monologues. A thoughtful pose. At the same time, the doctor leaned his head to one side and his eyes picked out different points in the room, a tactic he used perhaps because of the news he had to deliver or perhaps because it helped him to recall what it was he had to say. Whatever his reason for this annoying habit, I remember wishing he would look at me.

Yet over time I would come to appreciate his quirky mannerisms. And in spite of my initial impressions, he turned out to be attentive and professional. What I liked about him best was his wry sense of humour and the fact that he was bluntly honest. He wasn't negative or discouraging, quite the opposite, but he refused to promise something he couldn't deliver. Like most stroke survivors, I was searching for a miracle cure, a quick remedy, but rarely is there a quick or easy fix for a damaged brain.

The physiatrist introduced himself and told me how I was to address him. He wanted to be known as "Doctor" or "Doctor So-and-So." Nothing else would be acceptable. As insistent as he was, his title meant nothing to me, not out of any disrespect I felt towards him, but because what he had to say, the content of his message, mattered far more to me than any hospital code of conduct. Or label.

He was there, he said, to confirm officially that I had indeed had a stroke. I wanted to tell him that this was no longer front-page news. At least I didn't think so. By this time I think everyone, except me, was operating on the assumption that I had suffered a "brain attack." I found it weird, if not a tad unsettling, that this "official" diagnosis had taken so long to trickle down to me, the patient.

At first, he continued, they had thought my stroke fairly mild. Nothing had shown up on the initial CT scan, but a second scan had revealed something much more significant. And serious. I had suffered an ischemic stroke on the left side of my brain in the pons, a part of the brain stem. In other words, as a result of what they had now detected, I had "suffered fairly dense paralysis of the right upper extremity and distal lower extremity." His words.

My words: My right side was paralyzed, fact; I couldn't move, fact; my body ached, fact; and my speech was impaired, listen.

"What caused it?" I asked, my tongue still thick, my words muffled.

"We don't know. If I was to hazard a guess, and that's all it would be, I'd say hypertension. Your blood pressure was very high. But you have other conditions that could well have been contributing factors."

I knew this. I wanted to cry, but I wasn't going to let that happen. When I was a kid, six or seven, back on a school playground, I had been ridiculed for wearing shorts by an older boy, a bully who had pushed me to the ground and pummelled me as I cringed under his blows. I wouldn't cry then and I wouldn't cry now. My God, what punishments and mindless actions we tolerated to hold on to our innocence and self respect.

Again I started to replay my feelings of guilt. I was also incredibly weary and, for the first time, I was ready to admit that my thoughts had crossed into a remote place where life seemed cruel and without pleasure. And without pleasures, far too numerous to name, what was left? Without at least food, wine, song, story and sex, it was a dark, dark place, to be sure. My age, my health, my mortality, had become realities. It was me I saw in the mirror every morning, not some other older guy. I suppose my feelings at that moment had something to do with the doctor's confirmation that I had suffered a stroke. Perhaps until that moment I still held out hope that I had simply been knocked out by some form of a virulent virus — more denial — but that was not the case and I had to deal with it.

"The good news," the physiatrist said, "is that a bed has come available in rehab. Normally we keep stroke patients in acute care for about three weeks, followed by a couple of months in therapy, but if the rehab team is agreeable I'd like to move you to the rehab unit sooner, perhaps as early as Friday. I think you're a good candidate for our new program. We think the faster we can move patients back home and back to community living the faster they'll recover. You'll be put on a six- to eight-week intensive rehab course, followed by eight weeks, equally demanding, as an out-patient. You need to be committed and willing to work hard. What do you think?"

He wanted me to be a guinea pig. And I was more than happy to accommodate him, anything to escape my roommate and the noisy, crowded fourth floor where I felt like a cadaver in waiting.

"Yes, I can do it," I answered, although at that very moment my body suggested otherwise. Everything I couldn't move ached.

The prospect of returning home to my own bed was comforting and I knew I would finally get fed. The timing issue I hadn't quite resolved. Such calculations belonged to another universe.

"Yes," I repeated, "definitely. Count me in."

"Okay, we'll see what we can do. I'll let you know when we're ready to make the move."

Both Pat and I were delighted, Pat so much so that I think she thought I would be fully recovered within a few months. Later that night she wrote an email to family and friends that expressed her guarded optimism.

November 21, 2012

Hi all,

Just a note to let you know that Ron seems to have plateaued (is this a word?) and is possibly starting to make some strides forward. He did, e.g. today begin to dictate his Declaration of Dependence and suggested he and Stephen Hawking go on a speaking tour together. His mind is good. His right side is not so responsive. More tests are scheduled.

Ron might, however, be a good candidate for the rehab ward, which is excellent news. He would have to get the OK from "the team" for that. Having a house which is wheelchair friendly is all to the good here. In the meantime, Ron still has to pass the swallowing test so that he can get real food. The hospital is, of course, very crowded. Beds, equipment, and staff etc. all in the very crowded hallways.

Nicole is here for a day or two or three. Ron was thrilled to see his daughter.

Will write again tomorrow. Thank you for all your good wishes.

Love,
Pat

Little did we know.

In retrospect, Pat's unbridled optimism was premature. The reality was that early on neither of us had the slightest appreciation of how much determination and commitment was going to be necessary for the struggle ahead. We knew nothing about strokes — the enduring and uncompromising pain, the loss of self. And I, in my woeful ignorance, had no idea how dependent on others I would become.

Stroke recovery is a lengthy process, filled with many hidden surprises and mysteries for which there are no names. The severity of my stroke was still an unknown, as was its cause. The fate Pat and I were about to share would take us from euphoria in one moment to despair in the next. There was no room for indifference.

FIVE

A Mind in Mutiny:
Holding on through Memory

Although I had spent the past forty-eight hours flat on my back, I felt exhausted, as if I had just completed a triathlon. I don't know why I make this comparison. I'd never in my life run, cycled or swum any great distance, but the few times I'd watched competitors cross the finish line in such races on TV they'd always looked wrecked, much as I felt now. Why was I feeling this way? Perhaps because living in a mental state of anticipation can be far more tiring than any form of physical exertion for eight straight hours. Such physical toil — swinging an axe, raking asphalt or digging with a shovel — can make even the strongest and fittest body feel muscle weary. But this was different. This was mental fatigue. My brain felt as if it had been kneaded out of shape, not into shape. Promises or expectations, like dreams of partial or total recovery, demand tireless concentration and consume enormous reserves of energy. And persistent fears and anxieties, such as the possible onset of paralysis, or loss of memory or loss of identity, will invariably gnaw away at whatever brain cells have survived.

No wonder I wanted to bury my head in a pillow and seek refuge under warm covers.

With Pat and Nicole sitting on either side of the bed, I closed my eyes, not so much to sleep but to see if I could unscramble the mass of messages I was receiving from my body, my brain and from everyone who occupied the world out there, the world to which I no longer felt I belonged. As happy as I was to have Pat and Nicole at my side, I had other, more pressing matters to think about.

I was worried that no one knew the reason or reasons for my stroke. After all, without this knowledge how were they going to treat the symptoms and the illness? Or was a stroke, technically speaking, an illness? The part of my brain that had died as a result of the stroke was dead, not ill. Therefore, I decided, it was illness or neglect that had led to the stroke. My mind circled like a runaway twister. So the symptoms had to be the illness and the stroke the payoff. Or the forfeiture. I had earned my stroke! The good old-fashioned way.

And yet the question still banged away in my head, kept coming back, wouldn't go away. What had caused my stroke?

No one knew the cause with absolute certainty, least of all me. The experts have compiled a list of risk factors. These include high blood pressure, diabetes, high cholesterol (the bad type, LDL, although David Perlmutter, a neurologist, in his fascinating book, *Grain Brain*, argues that the brain thrives on cholesterol), sleep apnea and being overweight. Take your pick; I qualified on all of these fronts. A lot of us do, especially in North America. And these risk factors combined with ageing are a dynamite formula for cardiovascular and cerebrovascular problems of all sorts. My only question was why it had taken so long for me to have the big event? I had indulged myself and a host of bad habits for far too long. Granted, on the advice of my once-upon-a-time Scottish GP who had died of a heart attack at fifty-eight, I had played golf regularly for years; and I had coached youth soccer for eight years. But I had also smoked heavily until 1984, I had over-eaten for as long as I could remember, my jobs which I loved were sedentary and could be stressful, and I was overweight. Therefore, *why* I'd had a stroke was not a big surprise. If I'd known anything about stroke, I'd have nominated myself as a prime candidate. Maybe, and I like to think this is the case, if I'd been better informed, I would even have done something about it. On the other hand, I belong to that breed most likely to say "that'll never happen to me."

Now I wanted to make sure it wouldn't happen again. I was assuming that for the time being all the medications that were being pumped into me would prevent any immediate recurrence of a stroke. The prospect, moreover, of being moved to rehab so promptly where "The Team" would get me onto my feet and whip me into shape lifted my spirits enormously, along with the anti-depressant drug every stroke patient is prescribed. I think at the outset I was given at least ten different medications, not including the IV which was likely a concoction of electrolyte solutions, other medicines and nutrients. As I lay there mulling over all this information as best I could, I decided I wanted to wean myself from too much dependence on drugs as soon as I was able to do so. I was already experiencing one of the uncomfortable side effects of taking a combination of drugs: serious and increasingly painful constipation. This would become a major issue just before my departure for rehab.

Meanwhile Pat and Nicole chatted away, their voices running together like a creek surging during spring runoff. They had so much news to catch up on, especially about Flora. Stories were told, schoolyard stories, about encounters with older, worldly-wise children of four and five. Flora, at three, was all ears, and recently, responding to a dare, had fallen and scraped a knee. She'd cried, Nicole said, but after a little comforting she had worn a band-aid over her "owie" like a medal.

Nicole gave a rundown of a new contract she had signed with a First Nations band on the west coast of the island, something to do with a sewer line travelling through the site of a possible midden or burial mound; and Pat gave her version of what had transpired with me over the past forty-eight hours.

Was it really only that long? I didn't think so. I had found new ways to measure time: by pain, by memories, by the effort it took to move a toe or finger, by fear and the fragility it exposed. Ironically, time was no longer quite so remorseless; it seemed more a matter of a state of mind, or perhaps of heavenly bodies, like so many wheels, turning and returning.

As I hovered between sleep and wakefulness, I listened to their conversation navigate the subject of stroke in general, mine in particular. As they talked over and around me, neither of them could believe that this had happened to me. But then, neither could I. The wound, the invisible wound; the broken brain, the broken soul, the broken spirit; being unable to move; the endless tears; loss of self; all had descended on me with the force of a cataclysm. The unexpected, whether tinged with joy or sorrow, inevitably brings disbelief, I thought, and sometimes the enormity of such events can leave us speechless. The Holocaust, Palestine, genocide committed in Darfur, Cambodia, Uganda, Rwanda, Bosnia, Iraq, Mexico, Syria, take your pick, the list was so terribly long . . . so many sad, sad events about which we were relatively silent. Beside these atrocities my stroke paled.

Thoughts and images cycled into my brain at will, with no regard for time, place or content. The sight of a gull riding the air currents outside the hospital window triggered the brief flash of a stormy trans-Atlantic voyage Pat, Nicole (who was only two at the time) and I had made from Montreal to London aboard the Polish liner, the *Stefan Batory*, in 1977. While I sat in a bar, Pat took on the challenge of playing chess against a Dutch Grand Master who in his day-to-day life was a mathematician. He had been on sabbatical as a professor at the University of Michigan and was on his way home to Amsterdam. Pat lost three quick games, although to be fair she had almost won the third. One wrong move and he had pounced.

Where had we left Nicole? There must have been a babysitter on board the ship, a member of the crew. What a thing to forget. Vaguely, I remember a barren white room with bright blue carpet and plastic toys, illustrated books, a rocking horse, Lego blocks and rubber balls. I recall seeing a massive greenish-grey swell, the open Atlantic, through a porthole. Up and down we plunged.

I realize now that I was one of the lucky ones. Even though I was in a stupor, I could think and I could remember events, not just from earlier in the day but from different moments in my past. Later, other stroke survivors would tell me that, during the first days after their stroke, they couldn't remember the last thing they had done or said, let alone events from the past. From day to day they drew blanks. Each day was new and bewildering. Most alarming, they said, were the moments when, with their good arm, they would grab something scary and squirming in their bed that they didn't recognize and try to fling it onto the floor. Only then did they discover "it" was attached to them, the "it" being their own paralyzed arm or leg. One said he was certain he had grown a third arm. It was stuck under him and he couldn't get away from it. He had been terrified. He didn't know he was lying on his own paralyzed arm.

As I say, I was lucky. Even though I was paralyzed, I had my mind. And while I didn't know that "losing my mind or identity" was a possible side effect of a stroke, I was determined to hold on to what I had left.

My roommate was beginning to stir for the first time since lunch. He was emerging from his cocoon of sleep. He had already called for the nurse twice and was disgruntled because no one had responded. Huffing and puffing, every few minutes he muttered "shit" or "fuck," as if he were trying to thread a needle. Or maybe he thought obscenities would provoke an action that would change his circumstances, perhaps free him from the bondage of the bed.

As I've said before, hospitals are a form of improvisational theatre. They are busy, busy places and, as a patient, no matter what your wishes, you are a member of the cast. At any moment you can get swept up in the action. Between visitors, who are like a freelance audience, and hospital personnel, who are often all reading from different scripts, the place can be chaotic. If you're not the centre of attention, if you're not the main act at any particular moment, you're waiting in the wings to make your appearance, to take your turn in the spotlight. Everything going on around you is grand theatre. You're essential to the production, but you have to wait for your cue.

The place has its own rhythms and you have to adapt. For myself, I tried to retreat into silence. My roommate, on the other side of the curtain, had his own idea of what adaptation meant.

I could hear him suck in air and begin to gasp. He was hyperventilating. He'd done the same thing on a couple of occasions the previous night. His breathing would build up until he was heaving, at which point I became absolutely convinced he was about to explode. One time I'd pressed my panic button, and when the nurse came running to attend to me, and I told her I'd called for him, she had rolled her eyes and told me to call only if I were the one having the emergency. She'd brought him a paper cup of water, though, which seemed to soothe him. I felt vindicated. The ensuing silence was golden and I think I managed to catch a few minutes of sleep.

Soon I was sure he would start complaining that he was being neglected. Although I knew there was no one with him, he would mumble away in brief sentences about the sixth floor and give instructions about his water and juice. Apart from the parade of nurses who came at regular intervals to take and replace the vacuum bottle at the foot of his bed, he hadn't had any visitors. Slowly he would work himself into a frenzy. He wanted action and attention and he was determined to get it.

"Hello," he yelled.

He paused and I could hear him press his buzzer repeatedly.

"Hello, nurse." Pause. "Anybody there?"

He stopped again for a second, waited and listened.

Then he cursed.

"Where the hell is everybody? I've been abandoned and I'm dying of thirst. Help! I need fluid."

Outside, what little winter light there was lingered for a few more minutes, then the glass turned black and reflected a pale image of the three of us on the bed, mother, father, daughter, framed by the window. Our little tableau looking like a Renaissance painting, something you might expect to see painted on the walls in the Santa Maria della Scala (known locally and fondly as "the hospital") in Siena.

"Hello, on the other side of the curtain. Can someone help me? Sir, is that your daughter I hear with you? Can she fetch me some water?"

Nicole rose, as I knew she would, and said she would try to find a nurse, but just as she was about to step out a nurse came through the doorway.

"What can I do for you, love," she said to my roommate in a voice that sounded like the tinkling of bells.

How did she remain so cheery, I wondered? What a thankless job she had, attending to our endless demands and needs

"I'm marooned on an island of bedding," he said, "dying of thirst. Where is everybody? I've been pressing this damn buzzer and calling out for ages, but no one hears me."

"I heard," she said in a gentle voice, "I heard you. How could I not? But you're not my only patient, you know."

This rebuke had all the force of an apology.

"I came as fast as I could," she continued.

"I know, I know, I'm sorry," he said, attempting to sound contrite. "It's just that I'm so thirsty. You don't know — nobody knows — how thirsty I get."

"I think we do," she answered, "but more fluids really are your worst enemy."

Whatever restful mood had existed in the room suddenly dissolved. The painting in the window became harsh with a cold, otherworldly glare. It no longer depicted the portrait of a family in repose, gathered around a sickbed — what I assumed the traditional study of a consoling family would look like at the end of a master's brush. Instead it became utilitarian, functional, washed out. The mere reflection of a hospital room. A Polaroid photo perhaps.

What was it that made him so thirsty? And why did he have to harp on about it? I was annoyed.

Now that Nicole was standing, Pat had begun to gather up her things. Purse, puzzles, gloves, scarf, coat, keys.

"We've got to be going," she said, getting to her feet.

She straightened her back, a move I understood would not be contradicted.

"Must you?" I asked.

Placing the palm of her hand on my forehead, something she did when she thought I might have a fever, she caressed my right eyebrow with her thumb. She often did this just before we went out. She would lick her thumb and straighten out my eyebrows. Spit, but no polish, I thought. Over the years, I had been hopeless, a travesty of good grooming. Hairs sticking out every which way.

"Yes," she said. "As it is, we'll have to deal with rush hour. And you need to get some sleep."

How was I to sleep with him carrying on the way he did, I wanted to ask? I don't know what I expected. I knew she couldn't do anything about him and, even if she could, she wouldn't want to cause a scene. The simple reality was, I didn't want them to leave. Yet I knew how selfish my protests would sound, so I kept quiet. Pat had been with me since mid-morning, always attentive, always on alert. I was behaving like a spoiled puppy waiting to be petted. I had no right to try to wheedle favour this way. She'd already put in a lengthy shift.

As they slipped on their coats, I became overwhelmed by a crescendo of sadness. It seemed as though Nicole had just arrived, that we'd hardly spoken. Now they were leaving and I would be alone again. Where had the day gone? There is nothing quite like the moment of separation to magnify one's sense of loneliness and to stir a little self-pity, no matter how much one abhors it. Once again I wanted to weep, like a young boy waiting for the barber to give him his first haircut.

When hunger gets inside your head it's all you live for. Hunger persists. Consumes you.

Shortly after Pat and Nicole had left for the day, dinner was served. The smell of hot food wafted along the hallway and into our room. I hadn't eaten for three days and the fantasy meals I prepared for myself promised all sorts of taste delights. They had little to do with the plain food the hospital was serving to those who could swallow. My mind flirted with images of thinly sliced cuts of roast pork and beef, turkey, chicken, salmon, cod (which I preferred over halibut), roasted or baked potatoes (swimming in butter, chives and sour cream), carrots (preferably raw), beans, peas, spinach salad with pomegranate seeds and feta cheese, a dessert tray piled high with cakes, chocolates, wedges of lemon meringue pie, and soufflés.

If the only meal I was going to get was imaginary, I thought, I might as well write my own menu. And yet, I longed to meet the "Swallow Lady" who, with a little magic and a wave of her wand, would pronounce me fit to ingest food. And I would finally be able to go to sleep on a full stomach.

Next to me, I swore I could hear my roommate smack his lips, deliberately making slurping sounds, as though he were sipping soup or spooning up gravy. It sounded as if he was goading me. How could he possibly know about my hunger? Up and down the ward I could hear the kitchen staff collecting trays, which made me think more about my empty stomach and the swallow test I had to take the next day. What if I failed? How long could they feed me through an IV? When had I ever been this hungry? That was an easy question to answer. It had been in Paris at the tail end of the adventure that had taken me as far away as Gibraltar and Morocco. But it was on the road from Algeciras to Marseilles where my first experience of hunger had begun.

A few minutes later I had the nurse roll me on my left side and prop me up with pillows. Then I returned to northern Spain and my journey south, to my pockets stuffed with crusty rolls filled with delicious ham.

I was learning, as the long night began, that memories help you to find yourself, help you to reconnect with the person you seem to be losing. I was convinced that the more I could remember of my past the better my chances were of keeping in touch with who I was. Or with who I had been. With Pat's and Nicole's departure, everything was slipping away. Slip-sliding away — is this what Paul Simon's lyrics meant?

As I closed my eyes I found myself happily back in San Sebastián.

After we left the tapas bar our host dropped us off at a gas station on the outskirts of the city, on the main road leading to Madrid. A friend of his owned the station and our host suggested this was where we would have our best chance of thumbing a ride. The night continued cold and wet, and no one heading out of town at that late hour was willing to take a risk and offer a lift to two itinerant Canadians. Or perhaps they objected to the new growth on our faces, the longish hair and the musty smell we gave off after a few days on the road. We hadn't bathed since leaving London.

When we realized this is where we would spend the night, the attendant, using a crude form of sign language, suggested we take down stacked cardboard cartons of oil cans and form them into beds. We could spread our sleeping bags on top. At least this way we would be raised off the cement floor and away from the damp. Even so, I think this is the only time in my life I have ever suffered from anything resembling chilblains.

As I slept, shivering inside my sleeping bag, every so often I would hear the bell above the door jingle and a customer enter to pay a bill or purchase a coffee. Following the low hum of a brief conversation, there would be a sprinkle of good-natured laughter, followed by footsteps and the jingle of the bell again. So much coming and going with us half-asleep under the shop lights. I tried to imagine what they must be thinking and saying: *Where do you think they've landed from? Do you think they're on the run? What must their families think? Are they allergic to work? Both of them could use a good scrub and shave.* All the things my own parents would have thought and likely said had they seen us huddled in a corner like two stray alley cats.

Never mind, I thought, come morning we would begin our trek to Madrid, via Vitoria and Burgos. Then on to Malaga and the Mediterranean sun.

And warmth.

What I recalled from this point on, as I lay in my bed, came in fragments.

Between a nagging hunger, the continuing antics of my roommate and a pressing need for sleep, I forgot much more than I remembered. But the little I did remember fed my search for "me," although I had no idea at that moment of the extent of my loss. In a curious way, it was like building a house without blueprints. Each fragment of memory was a timber and, with each timber in its place, the structure began to take on a shape I could identify. The only problem was that there were important structural elements missing, like posts and bearing walls. Distinct rooms, a roof, ceilings, floors were all only implied by the pieces I was able to construct or remember. It was like an incomplete Escher drawing. But it was a start and it kept my brain occupied.

Our ride to Vitoria the next morning ended a kilometre or two before where the city proper began. Earlier in the day, as we climbed away from the coast, it had stopped raining, but a heavy cloud layer had pushed south with us and now hung over the buildings and streets of this stunning medieval town and gave them a greyish-brown, monochromatic appearance. After all these years, I remembered the walk into town vividly, for two reasons. This was when we ate the remaining ham-stuffed rolls. The bread was going stale, and it was the last of the food we had. So we ate thankfully. The second reason, which struck us both as incredibly bizarre, was that the beautiful, cobbled streets were empty. The shops were closed, the apartments seemed vacant, everybody appeared to have fled town, leaving a ghost city in their wake. Had we been thieves we could have opened doors and escaped with our bounty undetected.

It was eerie, as if a plague had passed through and no one had survived. Or it could have been the deserted set of a gothic movie about the Inquisition. Then we walked around a corner and a massive roar, a tsunami of sound, hit us. And then another wave. Somewhere ahead of us a crowd cheered with a single, excited voice, like the waves of sound one would have heard above the Colosseum during the peak days of ancient Rome. Only on this occasion it was in response to a football match, not to the excitement of gladiators doing combat or the replication of an historic battle with slaves sacrificed to ensure victory.

How did I know it was a football match? Now, when I thought about it, was I remembering Vitoria or Burgos? Or was I getting the two places mixed up? They had both been Roman settlements at some stage, I was sure of that. Then another memory edged into my mind. There were three girls, sisters, who had suddenly appeared in the street. Jim had asked them in French where all the people were and what the noise was. They had laughed and said, "*fútbol.*" Everyone in town was football mad, the eldest told us in broken English, and they're all at the game. Then the sisters invited us back to their apartment where, to our surprise, we were introduced to their mother and grandmother. They served us tea and cakes. Delicious and timely. It was the food I remembered, although I had the crazy sensation, both then and now, that we were being treated like prospective suitors.

Where, I wondered, had these memories been stored? And how much of what I was remembering bore any resemblance to the truth? I wanted to sleep, I was exhausted, I could feel my head sink into the pillow, but for some reason I felt compelled to know how much of my past I could reconstruct from these memories that had lain dormant for fifty years. Even with gaps in the narrative, I felt this was an encouraging sign that my brain was still working. Struggling to cultivate past memories was like pouring water on a neglected plant. With any luck, something would sprout.

I was hopeful.

Somewhere on the desert plateau between Burgos and Madrid, we stopped at a bar, a building with thick, earthen walls, a flat roof, a dirt floor and no windows. The counter, behind which the owner stood — was he grizzled or was I remembering a scene from a spaghetti western? — had been built with rough-sawn planks. The wine was heavy, almost chewy, I remembered, and, most importantly, cheap. A couple of bare light bulbs burnt overhead. So much for decor and atmosphere. I think the bar had been strategically placed in the middle of nowhere as a trucker's stop. Out of our dwindling funds we each bought a glass of what I suspected was the local "plonk." As zany as it seemed, we felt a need to celebrate having "almost" arrived in the heart of Spain.

Later that day, no more than an hour outside of Madrid by car, we trudged along the gravel shoulder, our heads down, collars up, fists buried deep in our jacket pockets, having given up on the idea of ever hitching a ride the final distance into the city. Occupants of cars that sped by had either stared straight ahead as if we were invisible or had made a concerted effort to examine some landmark on the horizon in the opposite direction from where we stood, thumbs out. Truckers had waved and honked their horns. They were in too much of a hurry to stop.

The temperature had been continually dropping and our worst fear was that we would be stranded in this wasteland after nightfall. With our knapsacks slung over our backs, we were resigned to walking the rest of the way into the Spanish capital. Then without warning, a pale-green car, an Opel, pulled off the pavement, scattering dust and stones. Three men turned and waved us on, urging us to jump in. Hesitantly, Jim opened the door and slid into the middle of the back seat. I followed him, not exactly grateful, as I should have been; I had an uneasy feeling in my gut, although based on what I couldn't say. Why had they stopped?

The two men in front, wearing well-groomed black mustaches, grinned broadly, and then jabbered away in a rush of Spanish as the driver pressed the pedal to the floor, and the tires spun as we fishtailed out onto the highway. Our friend in the rear seat offered us his hand, spoke softly what I assumed was a greeting, and then turned and looked out the side window. Disinterested or distracted, I didn't know which.

When the two in front realized we didn't understand a word they were saying, the one in the passenger seat twisted around and started to use hand gestures. He enunciated each of their names carefully, none of which I remembered, and then, pointing at our companion in the back, made horns with his index fingers. After performing this charade for several minutes, coupled with the injection of a little French and a lot of laughter, we finally figured they were trying to tell us that the fellow sitting next to Jim was a famous bullfighter and they were his managers. We were in luck, they said. We were in the presence of a famous Spanish personality.

"Royalty, he is royalty," they said in Spanish, "like the king and queen."

He turned from the window and told them to shush.

Jim smiled, nodded his head and said to me: "They must think we just got off the last boat. What's next?"

Would we like his autograph?

No, we were travelling light and didn't need anything more to weigh us down, I told them, my hands simultaneously weaving my message in the air.

When they saw we were doubtful they encouraged the bullfighter to show us his hand. Reluctantly he spread his left hand out in front of us. On one finger he wore a gold ring inset with the largest red stone I had ever seen. Presumably a ruby. In spite of this display, this gesture of assurance, we remained skeptical.

Half an hour later and after an awkward silence, we were in Madrid, and as suddenly as they had stopped to pick us up, they stopped and dropped us off. Ushered us out of the car with hasty, back-handed gestures. They were clearly upset that we hadn't been taken in by their little sideshow. The foreigners were too worldly-wise, I assumed they were thinking. On the other hand, I felt re-lieved as I watched their car disappear into the city traffic. I don't recall what I imagined they might have been, possibly members of the Mafia, but I had visions of spending my remaining days chained in the hold of a rusty old tanker. I'd seen far too many B-rated movies.

We found a student hostel and bunked down for the night. The next morning as we set out for the Prado, one of Madrid's famous museums, we came on a kiosk plastered with posters advertising events happening throughout the city and other major urban centres. Opera, dance, theatre, art exhibitions, concerts. And there, staring us in the face was a full-coloured image, a full-figured por-trait, of our quiet companion from the back seat of the Opel. He was posed, standing in the centre of Seville's Plaza de Toros de la Maestranza, probably the oldest and most famous bullfight arena in the world. I stood there gawking. Astonished. And disappointed, hugely disappointed, that I'd been so distrustful. He was the legiti-mate thing: a genuine *torero*. In the gold-embroidered suit of the *matador de toros* he looked invincible, not at all like the withdrawn figure huddled into the corner of the rear seat of the Opel. I remembered wondering at that moment how many more of these missed opportunities would I have in my lifetime.

John Berger writes: "The number of lives that enter our own is incalculable." This statement occupies the centre of an entire page in his *Here Is Where We Meet*. Before and after my stroke it is an idea to which I have given considerable thought because of its simple truth. And staggering implications. Included in that number are those who will brush up against us briefly and move on, and those who will perhaps alter the course of our lives and have a permanent place in our consciousness.

"Why are you in here?" I heard my roommate ask.

"Me? Are you asking me?" I slurred.

"Of course I'm asking you. Is there anyone else in the room?"

I wasn't prepared for his question.

"I've had a stroke," I answered, encouraged by his sudden interest. Perhaps, I thought, now that he knows what's happened to me, he'll leave me alone to rest. To sleep. To carry on with my travels.

"Oh, that's not good at all," he said. "Not at all. Bad, from what I know. Are you paralyzed?"

"I think so."

I hesitated.

"I'm still not sure. It might be temporary," I added slowly, pronouncing each syllable as carefully as possible, as if I were reading out of a primer.

"Oh, yes," he said, "you could be right. That's possible. I hope so."

At the time I remember wishing he had said this with more conviction.

I knew then that he wanted me to ask about him.

"What about you?"

"Ascites," he said. There was a short silence and then he continued, "It's okay, most people don't know what it is. I have a liver problem. A slight plumbing malfunction. I'm unable to get rid of fluids in the normal way. That's why I'm always so thirsty. I know it doesn't make any sense. But trust me, I'm always thirsty. They don't understand."

For a moment he was silent.

"I have about two hundred pounds of fluid retention crushing me. Sometimes I think I'm going to suffocate."

"No."

"Yes," he said. "I'm normally a small man but right now I weigh over three hundred pounds. I have the equivalent of two bags of cement sitting on top of me."

I tried to visualize what he was saying but I simply couldn't. I'd never heard of such a thing.

"That's what you see the nurses doing at the foot of the bed. They're removing fluid from me a litre at a time. But they can't do it fast enough. That's probably why they keep the curtain between us closed; they don't want you to see me."

"No," I said, "I'm sure it's in-tend-ed for pri-va-cy."

"No," he said, "it's because I look grotesque."

And he began to sob.

Quietly.

Gently.

He didn't want me to hear him.

I shouldn't have listened.

Of all the paintings in the Prado, three have never left me. Hierony-mus Bosch's *The Garden of Earthly Delights*, with its time-ticking narrative about what happened to men and women after they demanded free will. And got it.

On the left, we see the temptation of Adam and Eve in the garden, and then in the centre of the triptych, in the largest panel, we're treated to an erotic feast of sex, food and drink. Only to be followed on the right by an eternity in Hell. What a price Bosch felt we would have to pay for our first fling as free spirits; for our little flirtation with pleasures the church viewed as sinful. As packed as the painting is with temptations, with its bulging ripe fruits, with its totally bizarre imagery, I have never felt guilt in front of this fanciful vision. Only joy.

But it was in Goya's *Saturn Devouring His Son* that I saw the truly dark side of the human imagination. Goya, who died of a stroke at age eighty-two, spent four of the last ten years of his life decorating the interior walls of his own house with his "black paintings," those disturbing visions of an old man who must have felt inept, impotent and angry. What frightful nightmares they were. These paintings embodied the grotesque. Here, in their presence, I felt self-conscious. Perhaps he finally grew weary of painting those who held uncompromising power.

When I looked at *The Dog* and that vast unoccupied space the mutt stared up into, I couldn't begin to imagine the despair Goya must have felt. How lost he must have felt. How lonely and without hope.

As I lay in my bed, wedged between pillows and staring out the window, I knew Goya's was an empty place I didn't want to visit.

For the moment, our room was relatively silent. My roommate was still there, I could hear him breathe, but in a curious way it felt like he had gone. Like he was absent. If only momentarily. Perhaps his whimpering had embarrassed him, although it needn't have; I was learning quickly that tears keep us connected to our humanity.

SIX

The Swallow Lady

After my stroke, a lot was done to help me with the physical side of recovery, but little was done to assist me with the mental challenges, largely because no one knew what was happening inside my head. *I* knew my brain had been bombed in some way, but the best the medical profession could do was show me a scan of the bleed or the block. An aerial map. Mountains and rivers. Cities and farms. Otherwise my stroke was a total mystery, to them and to me, the patient. There were no intricate details. None of the tools of daily survival. Facing this large unknown was terrifying, for me as well as my family. No one could track the journeys I took or know the connections I'd lost or trace the thoughts that had plunged me deep into a sea of despair and longing. Normalcy, whatever that is, would have been a blessing.

Some stroke survivors face the fear of a mind possibly erased, while others contend with what seems to be a mind in mutiny. I recognized things I couldn't name and often I spoke a language no one else could understand. I understood; they didn't. Not to be intimidated, a pall of silence fell over me and I lived either through memories or in a closed world that orbits a different sun. I felt as if I were caught in a space between dimensions, a place where no one else had ever been.

The question was how to reconnect?

Joshua Foer in his fascinating and entertaining book, *Moonwalking with Einstein*, writes:

> But how exactly a collection of cells could "contain" a memory remained among the deepest conundrums of neuroscience.
>
> For all the advances that have been made in recent decades, it's still the case that no one has actually seen a memory in the human brain. Though advances in imaging technology have allowed neuroscientists to grasp much of the basic topography of the brain, and studies of neurons have given us a clear picture of what happens inside and between individual brain cells, science is still relatively clueless about what transpires in the circuitry of the cortex, the wrinkled outer layer of the brain that allows us to plan into the future, do long division, and write poetry, and which holds most of our memories . . . the brain makes sense up close and from far away. It's the in-between — the stuff of thought and memory, the language of the brain — that remains a profound mystery. (34)

As the evening hours dragged on, I became increasingly conscious of the limitations of my body. Movement seemed to take more and more effort. After lights-out on the ward was called, each minute seemed interminable. My mind became hyperactive. I caught a glimpse of a clock in the hall and started watching the second hand jerk its way from 1 to 12. A robotic movement. Sixty stutter steps to a minute. And I watched and listened to every one of these, mesmerized.

Fatigue continued: my body felt utterly exhausted, with the sort of weariness that envelopes you after you've completed a long list of duties, arduous tasks that need to get done but seem to have no purpose and bring no sense of fulfillment. And cause no physical complaint. The word "chores" comes to mind. Or perhaps they're jobs that come with a heavy load of responsibility but bring no joy, no satisfaction. Such tasks are onerous and tend to leave you feeling hollow. Overtired. No matter how weary you feel, sleep is impossible. You fret, toss and turn, the sheets get tangled and you beg to be released into oblivion.

Is it worth fighting? What for? As a kid, I remember being told the material value of one human body is a few cents, under a dollar, although these days it costs a lot to die. The price of inflation.

In my youth I had worked at my share of mindless jobs. Once, while working my first union job in a pulp mill, I was assigned to help one of the full-time labourers hose down the inside of a cement bunker where they mixed concentrated sulfuric acid for use in the pulp digesters. When we got on top of the massive cement cubes that held the acid, I noticed that one of the many pipes zigzagging across the space above the bunker had developed a slow leak, releasing a small, clear teardrop about every thirty seconds. I remembered examining the spot where the drip had eroded the concrete. Very slowly, a perfect saucer, the shape and size of a Frisbee, had been eroded into the surface of a two-foot-thick wall of cement.

Dressed from head to toe in a rubber suit and wearing a heavy-duty respirator mask, looking every bit like a figure out of *Star Wars*, I was asked to climb down a ladder inside the cube to spray down the walls. Stupidly, like a beast harnessed to a plough, I did as I was told. Even though I was wearing a mask, I lasted less than five minutes before the fumes began to overpower me. The "old hand" who had been doing this job for a couple of years managed to stay down for fifteen minutes. Even though we were supposed to spell each other off, I refused to go down the ladder a second time. Had the foreman heard about my refusal I would have been fired on the spot.

Later, over coffee, I discovered that my co-worker, who looked to be in his sixties, his skin as dry as rice paper and terribly wrinkled, was actually in his early thirties. He told me the guy who had done the job before him had slipped and fallen into six inches of acid, and by the time they scrambled down to pull him out there was at most ten pounds of him left to retrieve. Whether this claim was hyperbole or not, why do we take these risks? More significantly, why are we asked to take these risks?

A few days later, on my way into the plant, I stopped to help a man outside the mill's chemistry lab lift upright a half-full, fifty-gallon oil barrel. Just as the barrel reached the point of standing, he let go of his side without warning and my right hand was smashed between the rims of two barrels as the one we had lifted catapulted ahead and then wobbled back and forth into place.

After this "mishap" I was given a push-broom and told to sweep a length of road over which chip trucks delivered sawdust all day to the four giant, five-storey digesters used in the initial process of mixing pulp for the making of paper. My crushed hand was bandaged and useless.

Sweeping was a make-work project. On the road to the pyramids of sawdust, I'd get about fifteen feet of pavement swept, using my one good hand, before the next chip truck passed by trailing a new carpet of sawdust. When some of the drivers passed me by they shook their heads and smiled in disbelief. I swept the same fifteen feet of road for several days until the union went out on strike, and the company used the opportunity to get rid of me without having to worry about workman's compensation. I was too "green" to file a complaint. That work was laborious and brought on nights of restlessness. I agonized over the injustice of it all. I didn't yet know my rights; I only knew to howl at the moon.

Images from this brief stint in the pulp mill often come back to me; now as I lay there in my hospital bed fifty years later, I recalled that after I heard the gruesome story about the worker who fell into the acid, I hadn't been able to sleep for days. Was it nightmares about falling that kept me awake? Or was it a growing awareness of some of the terrible jobs we find ourselves doing; and concern about why things are the way they are? These events from the past merged with the moment, became a part of a continuum that helped feed my recovery.

As I took stock of everything that had happened to me over the past seventy-two hours, I knew I'd done nothing except lie on my back. Why was I so tired? It didn't make sense. Nothing added up. Entranced, I watched the second hand circle around the clock face yet again; I was like a kid viewing a peep show. Round and round it went.

As far as I could remember, a quick tally of what I had done throughout the present day looked like this: Pat and Nicole had taken turns pampering me; a woman had come twice from the lab to take several vials of blood; a nurse had taken my blood pressure and temperature on at least four different occasions; I had swallowed, yes swallowed, at least a dozen pills; my drip bag had been replaced; cleaning staff had breezed in and whisked the room and scrubbed the bathroom; my bed had been made, with me in it (I didn't think they had changed the sheets, although I couldn't swear to this); some woman had come to rent me a TV and phone, neither of which I could use because I had the attention span of a gnat; and I still couldn't speak well enough to make myself understood. I was worried that my bowels no longer seemed to be working. I was becoming obsessed about this potential blockage problem. And, if my bowels did work, how was I going to make it from the bed to the bathroom in time? Furthermore, what would happen when I pressed my buzzer in earnest?

I had done nothing, nil, zip, and yet I was oh, so weary. After all this inaction, without even working up a sweat, I felt totally whacked. Perhaps it was all the unknowns I had to worry about that were bearing down on me. When the body and brain reach the breaking point, adapting to change becomes a struggle. Once the brain's broken, how do you repair it? What if an overhaul were impossible? What if the stroke was fatal? If they hadn't been able to put Humpty Dumpty back together again, what were they going to do with me?

Next I wondered what sort of tortures awaited me. What exactly did the swallow tests entail? I imagined stainless steel instruments being used to trigger and test my gag reflex. I visualized a miniature camera on the end of some sort of probe being lowered down my throat. A catalogue of medical instruments, even from this technologically advanced world, still looked primitive, especially when viewed through an enhanced and terrified imagination.

I longed to escape. And to accomplish that I needed my roommate to keep up his new, albeit unstated, vow of silence. The only trace I could see of him now was the vacuum bottle at the foot of his bed. He had become a ghost. I couldn't even hear him breathe. It was so quiet on his side of the curtain that I became concerned he might have died on me. Or did he just want me to think that? No, no, I thought, he wasn't that clever or subtle. He would, I was certain of this, have had some parting words for me, some advice regarding my never giving up, organ donorship — in his case either a used kidney or liver, which he needed desperately — the politics of healing, or a rant about his latest conspiracy theory.

For the moment, though, I closed my eyes. In that delicious hush that had fallen over our room, I began to worry. My memories about my first trip to Europe were filled with increasingly bigger gaps. Perhaps my brain was more damaged than I was willing to admit. Or was this normal? After all, it had been fifty years since I'd had the impulse to reconstruct these events in such detail. Under normal circumstances was memory more like a slide-show or movie, selectively edited for highlights, than the presentation of a continuous narrative? Either way, I suppose, everything I was imagining could have been an invention. Perhaps that's what memory was.

Madrid was a vague image at best. What I remembered were block after block of narrow grey streets, walk-ups in five- or six-storey brick or granite buildings, ornamental tiles everywhere, the spectacular palace, Gran Vía Avenue from Plaza de España to Plaza de Cibeles, the Prado and parks. At its heart, Madrid was a pretty city. But it was colder than Paris, not at all what we had expected. And the one cooked meal I'd eaten off a menu written in Spanish that I couldn't translate, octopus prepared in its own ink, had turned my stomach, not because it wasn't tasty but because of what it was. If only I hadn't insisted the waiter describe what I'd just eaten. He used his fingers to convey an image of the octopus moving through water. I excused myself from the table, stepped out back and wretched. I already knew the power of the imagination.

A couple from the hostel, who owned an old VW van, was heading south and Jim asked if we could tag along. I tried to remember the couple and the journey, but all that came to mind was a huge blank; they were less distinctive than the stick figures in a child's drawing, and the rolling countryside through which we travelled was unremarkable. All I could rummage up were endless rolling sienna-coloured hills — rocks, tufts of grass and dust — dotted with scruffy, prickly looking trees. Ilex or holm oaks. A badlands into which spaghetti westerns easily fit. There might have been the odd olive grove, but then, when I thought about it, they might have belonged to another trip to Spain, viewed through a train window, and in a different region of the country altogether, at a much later date — when my daughter was living in Madrid, teaching ESL, and we had made a trip to Barcelona to view the magical constructions of Antoni Gaudi.

As we crossed the plateau in the van, occasionally we came across small buildings perched on the sides of hills, often surrounded by drystone walls, possibly enclosures for sheep or goats. For the most part, this largely horizontal landscape was harsh and arid, a quiet reminder that there are places in this world indifferent to life.

Lurching and swaying like an overloaded pack mule, the VW made a descent of what seemed like several thousand feet on a narrow switchback road, no wider than a goat track — I'm sure this is an exaggeration and the road was at least the width of a car — brakes scraping, down to Malaga, a small white-washed city far below that hugged a bay on the edge of the sunlit and sparkling Mediterranean Sea.

And then on we went to Gibraltar. Past Torremolinos and Marbella.

But why? Why had we done that?

For the life of me, I couldn't remember why we had bypassed Malaga and headed straight for a landmark that in classical mythology was known as one of the Pillars of Hercules. I was surprised by how readily this name jumped to the front of my mind. Once again I marvelled at the amount of information I had stored away in my brain and how quickly I could access those files. I wondered if that information had a stale date. Or had the stroke attacked my memory files? Our brains have an amazing capacity not only to retain information for future reference, but with a little effort they can sort out and deliver the most obscure — sometimes petty, sometimes profound — tidbits of data.

More recently, Gibraltar was simply referred to as the "Rock." How did I know that? I hadn't thought about Gibraltar in years. Perhaps it had cropped up as an answer in a TV quiz show or in a documentary or in a novel. Who knew? Memories seldom came with references. Some of the details, though, of that long-ago trip were surprisingly vivid. Then it struck me, the more plausible reason for continuing on to Gibraltar was simple: that's where our ride was going. Logic stepped in and filled in the gaps. My brain *was* working. I suddenly remembered that Gibraltar was where the young couple — I think they were Australians — were going; they had a boat to catch that would take them from Algeciras to Tangiers. Somewhat unceremoniously they dropped us off at the border crossing between Spain and Gibraltar and hurried on their way.

I was confused. Why was I trying to dredge up this fifty-year-old history? Then I remembered that it had all begun with my feeling hungry. I still felt hungry, famished in fact. I had heard the kitchen staff deliver all the other patients a bedtime snack. Once again I was not a part of the rotation. Nothing had changed. Before I could eat, I needed approval from the "Swallow Lady."

And that fateful occasion, when I had previously experienced the same sort of hunger I now felt, I knew had taken place in Paris. For some reason, I sensed I needed to take this journey to explain my present hunger. This all happened very rapidly. Each memory like a blink.

I realize now that I'm beginning to impose a chronology on my memories, a chronology that did not happen in "stroke time," if there is such a thing. Yes, I watched the clock move, that's true, but I'm not sure the passage of time meant much to me. In fact, I don't think it did. Not at all. Time was a part of that other world, the one outside of the room. Rather than a composition of things and actions, "now" was a mix of emotions, desires, indecisions, wishes and regrets. Recollections, when they came, were random. Associations helped me to reconnect to who I thought I might be; they provided me with the reassurance that I wasn't a stranger, even though the terrain I currently inhabited was unrecognizable.

Crossing from Franco's Spain into the British territory of Gibraltar took us at least two hours, perhaps longer. In 1965 Franco was engaged in a dispute with the Brits about the ownership of this barren, monolithic promontory of limestone, sandstone and shale at the foot of the Iberian Peninsula. He wanted the "Rock" for Spain. After all, it was attached to the Iberian land mass, and Spain's claim made sense, but the Brits invoked the Treaty of

Utrecht signed in 1713 as their deed to this small but very strategic "hollow mountain." It guarded the entrance to the Mediterranean and the shipping routes that led to the Far East via Suez.

Spanish customs officials rummaged through everyone's backpacks and suitcases, pretending to look for contraband, while several members of the Guardia Civil examined our passports, as if they expected to find someone wearing a disguise who was wanted by Interpol. All these men in different uniforms playing at security. Then, when they had been sufficiently annoying, prolonging a ritual that should have taken no longer than a few minutes, they released two dozen or so of us to wander across the airstrip that separated the two jurisdictions. We scampered across the tarmac, concerned that they might have timed our release with the arrival or departure of a plane. They looked that sinister in their three-cornered hats. If I remembered correctly the runway was one of the main roads of Gibraltar.

The town that sat at the foot of the "Rock" was insistently British, as quaint as the thruppenny bit, and undoubtedly intended to remind Franco not to try to tinker with the map. The Watney's pub we entered offered the same fare found on most chalkboards or menus back in the UK. Fish and chips, mushy peas, steak and kidney pie, shepherd's pie, bangers and mash, stew and hard, bubble and squeak, ploughman's lunch, roast beef and Yorkshire pudding. This was a menu spoken or read throughout the counties, from north to south.

After lunch, we began our ascent of the "Rock," climbing along narrow lanes and up worn stone stairs, past Barbary apes (actually tailless monkeys) sitting on stone walls and begging for food, past lovely gardens, towards the top of the mountain at just over four hundred metres. I had no idea why I was doing this. I was then, and still am, terrified of heights. As I lay in bed, motionless, and remembered the climb, I could feel shivers run through my limbs, and I sensed a weakness behind my knees that I invariably experienced when I viewed or imagined looking down from high in the air, whether from the top rung of a ladder or from an alpine path that wound its way along a ridge and provided a vista of distant farm fields and villages below. Recently I had started to feel vertigo even when I looked at moving pictures taken from a great height, in particular from gliders or balloons or paragliders. Movie shots taken looking down from the tops of buildings made me feel queasy and faint.

Now, as I journeyed back to Gibraltar, I was about to do something that made no sense, that was completely out of character.

As we reached a point two-thirds of the way to the top, we came to a road bordered on the upper side by a chain-link fence. Every fifty feet or so there were warning signs posted by some local military authority that read KEEP OUT. Naturally, for two young "adventurers" who felt they had the world by the tail, this was an invitation to scale the fence and explore. Inside, on the summit of the mountain, were a few small buildings, some low trees, shrubs and vines — honeysuckle and jasmine amongst them, I think — and what looked like radio towers of some sort. We weren't interested in those; we wanted to be able to say we had stood at the very pinnacle of Gibraltar.

I have no idea how I did what I did. I had taken several photographs of the water catchers on the eastern slope, looking straight down. And there were a few photos that presented a panorama of the Spanish and African coastlines in the distance. But it is the photos of the massive water catchers, used to collect rainwater, which baffled me. From all the prospects presented, it looked like I must have been straddling the mountain. Some form of trick photography had to be involved; I would never have been so brave.

I wonder now if it is the things we fear that we best remember. As I think about that moment atop Gibraltar, I realize that it is neither the height nor the falling I fear, but the temptation to jump. Is this a response to vertigo? And did the vertigo I felt then register in the same part of my brain as the vertigo that was a prelude to my stroke? How and why are the two connected?

In the weeks before I had my stroke, I had spells of dizziness, none of them in response to my fear of heights. Only months after the stroke did I recall them and think they might have had some significance. Why, I wondered, as I looked back on myself from the future, did I not see what were obvious warning signs? I would be standing or lying down and suddenly the room I was in would begin to do flips. It was as though part of me was operating like a gyroscope but without providing stability to the axis. Everything began to spin and spin, until I felt nauseated and the only way to gain relief was to shut my eyes. At the time I had simply dismissed these moments of disorientation as bouts of vertigo, something that happened to people as they aged.

Was this another warning sign that went unheeded?

Then one day, while out golfing, maybe three or four weeks before my life was rocked by the stroke, I stood on the ninth hole of our local course at the top of a hill, ready to take my second shot. I often played to this vantage point on this hole because it presented the best view of the pond, traps and green. What remained was an easy nine-iron shot to the pin. I swung and fell down. Straight down. My feet didn't slip out from under me, nor did I lunge forward; I just collapsed, at least I think that's what happened. The ground was wet and muddy and I assumed I had slipped. But in retrospect I had no recollection of how I fell. I took a swing at the ball and the next thing I knew I was staring at terra firma from as close-up as you can get. The end of my nose was wearing a piece of turf. My playing partner appeared at my side and offered to help me up. We laughed, but I had to admit I was shaken; there was a length of time, the duration of which remains unknown, about which I knew nothing. *Nada.* For all I knew, I could have spent a lifetime in another universe or dimension.

A friend of mine who had suffered a stroke ten years earlier had an identical experience a month or two before his major brain attack. He said: "Out of the blue, I collapsed, on the golf course. It was a hot day, one of those days when the air hovers above the earth like it does over a griddle, and I thought I had fainted from the heat. But later my GP told me I had probably experienced my first stroke."

Strokes are insidious. Like avalanches or tornadoes, they surprise their victims with their suddenness. Their stealth.

About three years after Jim and I visited Gibraltar, Franco tired of the squabbling and closed down the land bridge between Spain and the British territory, and it wasn't reopened until 1985, long after Franco's death. In the intervening years, if you wanted to tour the small town that sat at the base of the "Rock" or climb to the top for a view of Africa or were sent there for military reasons, you had to arrive and depart by sea or air.

After spending a few days in Morocco, visiting the Kasbah and other highlights of the Medina, we returned to Spain and hitch-hiked along the Mediterranean coast towards Barcelona. By this time, I was running low on cash, and I was constantly on the hunt for food, especially if it was free. In Malaga, orange trees laden with fruit grew down the centre of public boulevards and were ripe for the picking. As my arm stretched up into a tree, an old woman dressed all in black emerged like a crow from the shadows of a nearby building and scolded me. "*Público, público,*" she said, wagging her finger. In her other hand she held a broom. I don't believe in omens, but if I did she was certainly one I would have heeded.

As it was, I stuffed my pockets with fresh fruit, only to discover later the oranges were small and bitter. Probably marmalade oranges.

Just outside of Barcelona, on our way to Marseilles, we were picked up by a well-dressed man — pants neatly pressed, tie, jacket slung carefully over the back of the passenger seat — driving a large Mercedes. Quite plush. Opulent. For some reason it brought to mind Bob Dylan's "Talkin' World War Three Blues" in which Dylan was driving a Cadillac through the deserted streets of New York after an imaginary nuclear war, listening to his "Conelrad," a car radio. Yes, I thought, a Mercedes was the perfect cruising car for two vagrants bumming their way along one of the most expensive coastlines in the world.

"I'll let you be in my dreams if I can be in yours," Dylan sang.

Somewhere along this winding highway, in a small fishing village, the beach dotted with brightly painted boats — red, blue, green, yellow — I have no idea any more if we were in Spain or France, although I like to think we were in the small town where Salvador Dali grew up — our driver pulled off the road in front of a shop and told us he needed something to eat. Were we hungry? Could he get us something? We both nodded and smiled. Food at last. Perhaps a pastry or, better still, a sandwich. In the last few days all I'd eaten were bitter oranges. When he returned to the car he was carrying a small paper bag, hardly large enough to contain anything substantial. He handed it to us and told us to help ourselves. Inside was an assortment of candies and chocolate bars. I remembered my disappointment. I wanted to say to him, you drive *this* car and that's the best you can do? Sugar!

When I think about my response now, I'm surprised by my lack of gratitude, but then I was hungry, and a chocolate bar gave me nothing but a short rush of adrenalin. A tease. I'm once again reminded of how much hunger can undermine confidence and occupy and distort one's thinking. Frailty becomes desperation.

Meanwhile, Jim confided his new plans to me. He had decided to hitchhike to Islamabad. He had heard from someone back home that there were positions teaching English as a second language available throughout Pakistan. I was welcome to join him, he said. As tantalizing as the idea was, I explained I had only a few francs left and I had already wired home to have money sent to the American Express office in Paris. You can have it forwarded, he told me, but to be honest I was not thrilled about hitchhiking across the Middle East. It was too risky, I said. A landscape filled, at least in my imagination, with bandits, camels and sand. Besides, I told him, there's so much more of France and Europe to see.

Outside Marseilles, we parted company. Months later I would learn from his brother that Jim had made it safely to Pakistan's new capital and had found a job as an English instructor. Looking back, the direction I would take in my own life was a little less clear.

As hard as I concentrated I could not remember how I came to be sitting cross-legged on the verge of the main *autoroute* north from Lyon to Paris. How had I got from Marseilles to Lyon? For that matter, how had I got to the other side of Lyon? I was pretty sure I hadn't walked. I was simply too hungry and too weak to leg it any distance. For over two hours I sat with my thumb stuck out, despairing of ever catching another ride, when unexpectedly a small vehicle skidded to a stop inches from me.

Painted a powder-blue and dark green with large patches of rusty-coloured primer, the car I was looking at appeared to be an older model Renault. Bumpers, chrome, all unnecessary details had been removed from the exterior, as if someone had tried to disguise the make of the car. A large figure "8" was stuck on the door. I could hear the driver yelling, *"Vite, vite, montez vite!"*

As I stumbled to my feet the passenger door flew open, and when I looked inside I could see that with the exception of the driver's seat, the entire interior had been gutted, like a fish prepared for the frying pan. All that was left were frame and panels. In place of the passenger seat, there was a small wooden box which the driver flipped upside-down and directed me to sit on. Before I'd closed the door, we were gunning it back onto the highway. I remembered grabbing an edge of what had been the glove compartment and holding on for dear life.

Night sounds on a hospital ward are muted and tend to draw

attention to the invisible. Like a sign in a library, QUIET is written large on the world. It's what you can no longer see, though, that sticks out in your mind — all the things you once took for granted. Simple things like trees, birds, the sea, cloud formations, the sun, the stars, a full moon in a clear sky.

I must have been too quiet for too long, because a nurse carrying a flashlight came by to see if I was okay. She held my wrist lightly and took my pulse. Then she shuffled away into the night and I returned to my ride.

He drove like a maniac. Speaking a mixture of French and English, he told me I was now a participant in some sort of car rally. Our destination was the centre of Paris. He had lost precious time when he stopped to pick me up, not to mention my added weight, so — how do you say in English, he asked — hold on! We sailed around corners and took to the air whenever we reached the top of a rise. We bounded through the French countryside like a hare pursued by a fox. The sheer terror of it all was exhilarating. With the number on the side of the car there seemed to be no speed limit, even when we entered and were driving through the narrow cavernous residential streets of the old city. And then, in the early evening, we came to an immense, lighted square, filled with cars, a fountain and hundreds of people milling around. The car screeched to a halt, the driver revved the engine a couple of times — sound effects seemingly a part of the drama — and for the first time in a few hours the world came to a standstill.

Without the constant noise of the engine, tires and wind; without the blur of movement; without the constantly receding landscape — farm houses, fields, cows, horses, hedges, barns, trees, passed cars — there was calm. A blissful peace. For a moment we both sat and stared out the windshield.

I was in the heart of Paris, but in which district or arrondissement, I had no idea.

Then suddenly my new friend shook my hand and wished me

good luck. *"Au revoir. Bonne chance,"* he said and unbuckled himself from his seat. Only then did it strike me that I'd been sitting on a wooden box the size of a Japanese orange crate and he had been strapped in and wearing gloves and coveralls. I didn't and don't recall him using a helmet, but it wouldn't have surprised me if he had been doing so. That was it. As soon as he stepped out of his car he was surrounded by a crowd and embraced by a woman. His girlfriend? His wife? His lover? It didn't matter, I was forgotten. I grabbed my backpack, found a signpost, and began walking in the direction of the Gare du Nord.

I was starving, having not eaten a decent meal in three weeks, and I recalled a couple of inexpensive restaurants near the railway station. I had eight francs and a few coins in my pocket. Just over two dollars. Looking back, I realized it had probably been a blessing that I had been a passenger in the race on an empty stomach. But now I definitely needed food. And a place to sleep.

What happened next was unclear. My memory at this point was filled with doubts. Everything became muddled. I tried shifting my body, but only half of me would obey my directions. The bed was on an incline, which made movement more difficult. If I could only get into the right position, I told myself, my thoughts might settle, like sand on a seabed after a storm.

Movement and mindfulness seemed to me to be linked. In both senses, I had to find the right position. I don't know why I thought this. What I did know was the following: events were happening in three different times. There was memory in stroke time, memory in real time, and then there were the "facts" of historical time. I had no idea which was which. Presumably what had actually taken place had occurred during historical time, although I was well aware that there was no way I could know which was which with any degree of certainty. But that's what I hoped to resolve and get right. Likely what would emerge would be a blend of the three. I needed to accept the idea that ultimately memory was an invention, another reality. In order for me to find "me," I needed to sift through these variations of memory to arrive at something that at least resembled the historical truth.

Truth! Who was I kidding?

On and on my thoughts circled as if they had been arranged in a centrifuge. I decided that perhaps returning to the latest version of the story would help me focus. Confirmation that I wasn't losing my mind was becoming more and more pressing. I closed my eyes and slipped back into dreamland.

And instantly started to sort through a giddy maze of complex memories.

Like a stray dog I walked up and down a Paris sidewalk in front of a cafeteria-style eatery where menus were posted in a couple of windows. Moving from one menu to the next, I looked at the printed photographs of several of the meals. I stared through the window at plates of food sitting on the tables of other patrons: spaghetti, salads, veal cutlets with *pommes frites* and vegetables, pizzas, served with baskets of bread and glasses of wine. What a sight I must have been, or should have been, stalking the diners' meals, although to be honest I never had been one to worry about being spotted in a crowd. The best I could do with the money I had left was buy a plate of french fries, which would at least fill the empty space in my stomach.

While I waited for the restaurant to empty, I retreated across the street to the square in front of the massive stone facade of the Gare du Nord. This was where I had first arrived in Paris and for some inexplicable reason it was the one place to which I felt connected. Perhaps it was the long umbilical cord of familiarity stretching back to London that eased my mind. During our earlier stay, other landmarks — the Eiffel Tower, the Arc de Triomphe, Notre Dame, the Louvre, Montmartre, and the grand sprawl of the Champs-Élysées — had simply been points of destination from our hotel which was somewhere on the Left Bank in the Latin Quarter near the Sorbonne. I had no idea how to get there from where I was. Besides, I didn't have enough money to pay for a hotel. And at that moment, hunger trumped my need for shelter and a bed.

I found a cold bench in the night shadows and sat down. Looking longingly at the brightly lit windows of the restaurant, I imagined crêpes stuffed with cheese — Asiago, ricotta, Romano, provolone, parmigiano or mozzarella possibly — why was I suddenly thinking Italian — and vegetables cut as thinly as wafers floating in a white sauce, followed by a crème brûlée or fresh fruit.

When exactly the man approached me, I couldn't remember. Details chased after each other like a cat after its tail. Was it when I was sitting on the bench in front of the Gare du Nord? Or, was it when I moved to a table in the restaurant, where I recalled gobbling down a plate of french fries smothered in ketchup? He was dressed in jeans and a brown leather jacket worn over a blue turtleneck sweater. I remembered worrying that I was about to be hustled. This was the last thing I needed. He reached into his pocket and pulled out his wallet, and I prepared to tell him I wasn't his type. He had made a mistake, I would tell him, and turn my attention to the newspaper someone had left behind. I needed to practise my French. It was then I saw his Gendarmerie badge.

As we faced each other across the table, he asked me in a kind voice how I was doing and where I planned to spend the night. Much to my surprise he went on to tell me the restaurant would be closing at midnight, after all it was Sunday, and if I needed something perhaps he could help me. He knew the owner. He rose, walked over to the cash register and returned with a bun stuffed with something that resembled a hot dog, although it tasted nothing like any hot dog I'd ever eaten. My stomach immediately rebelled against the onions, but I think I would have eaten plaster or a paper plate with the right condiments.

I knew this encounter took place, but the sequence and what actually happened after was lost in a thick cloak of vapour or mystery.

When the restaurant closed its doors, he guided me back to the square, pointed to the same bench in the shadows I had sat on earlier, and disappeared. I will never know but I have always suspected that I had a guardian angel watching over me that cold, cold night in Paris.

The next morning, under a heavy grey sky, I was sitting on the cement stairs of the American Express office waiting for them to open for business. At no other time in my life had I felt so desperate. Nor, until I had the stroke, had I felt that way since. When the doors to the ornate building were unlocked and I stepped across the threshold, all I saw was an intimidating space with elegant columns, lofty ceilings and marble floors. I walked quickly up to a counter, made of richly milled mahogany, gave my name and showed whoever it was behind the counter my passport — I have no recollection if the person who answered me was male or female, spoke English or French, was short or tall, friendly or aloof — and turned away in disbelief, totally devastated, when I was told there was no letter or money transfer in my name.

Slowly I backed away, walked a few feet and collapsed.

I was exhausted and starving, much as I felt now in the warmth of my hospital bed. Wasn't this the reason in the first place for this stroll down memory lane — to remember in its cyclical complexity the similarities between that long-ago event and my present situation? Only back then I belonged to the outside world in which my body craved and needed nourishment, whereas now I was on a form of life-support being fed through tubes, was in considerable pain and had stared down the tunnel of time. And, much to my surprise, all those two events shared in common was an empty stomach. That was "me," I thought, an empty stomach, because I could link a distant memory to the present moment in a way that made both contemporary. Or was that coincidence, just another way we have of making order? Of connecting. Or disconnecting.

Which was *I* doing?

I tried speaking. Was I speaking in my memory or to someone in my room? And while I knew what I was attempting to say, once again the sounds I heard didn't quite match the thoughts I was having. In fact, when I listened carefully, the sounds made little sense. Why was this happening? Why couldn't I speak more clearly? I had to try harder. If I wanted to pass the swallow test and finally get fed, I was pretty certain I would need to have better control over my mouth and tongue. For some reason they weren't in sync with my brain. Nothing fit into my brain. I was in hospital, but in that moment I couldn't remember why?

I hurt, all over. Had I fallen? When I had seen my face reflected in the bathroom mirror I couldn't see any bruises. I couldn't remember falling. Why the pain then?

Pat had gone home.

With Nicole.

Outside it was pitch-black. The sky was starless.

Birdless.

Then I heard a man talking; on and on he went. My roommate. I remembered. As suddenly as the patter beside me had stopped it began. Around midnight. He was talking about Obama, the American president.

"He's no better than the rest of them. He intends to overthrow the middle class. They're all in cahoots, the whole lot of them. It doesn't matter which party you belong to, Democrat or Republican. They're all the same. It's what I was telling you earlier."

Earlier? What earlier?

"When we were talking about Kennedy. Do you remember?"

No, I thought.

"Yes," I said.

"Well," he continued, "those who have the money and the power will do anything to maintain the status quo. Including murder. Obama's totally tangled up with that Wall Street crowd. That's why he bailed them out. Along with the major automakers."

I let out a big groan. I didn't care. I wanted him to shut up. He had been peddling his conspiracy theories off and on for two nights. He had grown tiresome with his joyless and ponderous views of the world. He stomped out his ideas like he was trying to kill a household pest or put out a brush fire. When I tried to think about what he was saying, a baleful noise filled the precious silence in the back of my head. Everything he said seemed so senseless. QUIET, I thought. I wanted the silence you find when seated in a rowboat, in the middle of a lake, becalmed, with a cloak of stars overhead. Hadn't I read that Einstein conceived most of his grand ideas while floating on Lake Geneva? I wanted that moment when the pulse of the earth feels in harmony with one's own biorhythms.

Then I heard a woman speaking. Was she a nurse or was she from my memory?

"Are you okay?"

Kneeling down beside me, a woman helped raise me to my feet and into a nearby chair. Embarrassed, I stared down at the floor, not daring to look into her eyes, which if I had done so were a deep, soft brown. Everyone rushed around us, ignoring us, as if we were two boulders in a stream. All I could say was: "*Merci*," followed by a whimpering, "What am I going to do now?"

For the first time in my life, I was scared, truly scared. There had been things in the past which I didn't want to do or that were a challenge beyond my ability or willingness to do, but to those I had always had an answer. I had always been in control. But now, without money, I was powerless, something most of the world's population knew all too well. I was famished, but had no money for food; and I was exhausted and ashamed, with no place to go.

Then I took a quick glance at the woman who had helped me.

"I know you," I said, "don't I?"

"Yes, we met in Madrid, at the hostel." She held my hand, as if suddenly reunited with an old family member. "Have you a place to stay?"

"No," I said and hesitated. I didn't want her to know how desperate I was. It was a question of dignity. Yet I needed the help, pure and simple.

"No," I finally repeated, "not really."

"Then you'd better come with me."

We walked a few blocks, or so it seemed at the time, my mind filled with hallucinations brought on by hunger, to her small hotel, a five-floor walk-up with a reception area no larger than a pantry where she arranged for me to have a room. She also arranged for the older woman who ran the place to feed me for two days. Each day, three times a day, punctually, the old woman, her greying hair done up in a tidy bun at the back, her skirt ankle-length, her billowy blouse fulsome, knocked gently at the door, entered with a tray and served me a bowl of broth, a thick slice of bread, cheese, a piece of fruit and a glass of water. Otherwise I slept for well over forty-eight hours straight. A sloth waiting for his resurrection.

The American woman whom I'd met in Madrid saw me safely to bed, then she disappeared, not for just a few hours or for a day, but out of my life altogether. Gone. Forever. This Good Samaritan, this saviour, paid for my hotel room and my meals and left no forwarding address, no way for me to thank her.

I felt blessed, then and now.

Joshua Foer in *Moonwalking with Einstein*, writes: "In ways as obscure as sexing chickens and as profound as diagnosing an illness, who we are and what we do is fundamentally a function of what we remember." (67) That much I had begun to realize as a result of my memory trips through France, Spain and Morocco. I was certain these associations I was making were helping me to remember who I was, even though the journey, the shift from present to past and back, was often bewildering. But now, as I lay in bed, my memory most of all reminded me of the generosity and caring nature and spirit that sustains hope at the core of the human consciousness.

I fell into a deep sleep with my roommate reminding me that the moonwalks taken by Neil Armstrong and Buzz Aldrin in 1969 had been filmed in the deserts of Arizona or Nevada. I can't remember which.

The next morning, some time between nine and ten, not long after Pat and Nicole had arrived back on the ward to spend the day, a man and two women poked their heads around the corner of the privacy curtain.

"Mr. Smith?" the man asked.

I nodded and they squeezed into my half of the room, forcing Nicole to retreat into the hall. One of the women was pushing a wheelchair. Pat continued to sit on the one chair by the window. I was confident she wouldn't be budged.

"We've come to take you for a walk," one of the women said.

Good bloody luck, I thought. Just the mention of movement made me feel even more like a legless lump, like something you might see on exhibit at the carnival next to the bearded lady or the man with three legs and two sets of genitalia.

"And perhaps for a spin around the ward," the man continued, glancing back and forth between me and the wheelchair.

Oh joy, I thought, a spin around the ward, that'll be a treat. I was tempted to ask if it would be a time trial. His intentions were good, but I didn't want to move, I didn't want to see other sick people, and I was worried that I was going to be separated from Pat and Nicole. Since waking, when breakfast was served to the rest of the floor, I had been anticipating Pat's and Nicole's arrival. Increasingly, in what had become a totally unfamiliar world, my family was becoming my one constant, and I was horrified that I would lose the connection.

I didn't quite know what to make of this new threesome. They were all dressed casually, in running shoes and brightly coloured sweatsuits, and looked as though they had recently walked out of a jazzercise class where they danced to the same music that escaped from my roommate's earphones — some fusion of jazz and Lady Gaga.

They were so young, all smiles and jovial voices. In one sense I loved their enthusiasm, their obvious attempts at empathy, but deep down I knew there was no way they could begin to understand what I was going through. They were busy embracing life, like kites riding the wind currents, which was what they should have been doing, while I was lost behind a wall of uncertainty and distrust.

"We're physiotherapists. We've come to get you out of bed," the other woman said.

"Oh, have you?" I said, my voice once again sounding like I was speaking through a rubber dam.

"The faster we can get you up, the better we can assess your needs," the man said.

My needs, I wondered?

"For therapy," one of the women added.

"Yes, for therapy. We know from experience, the sooner we can get you moving, especially after a stroke, the better your chances for recovery," he continued.

Although I had managed to sleep for a few hours I was having difficulty opening my eyes and focusing my thoughts. Both seemed mired in sludge. Everything seemed dull around the edges and thick, like porridge. Perhaps it was the drugs, I told myself. Instead of feeling well rested, I felt like I'd spent the night hiking up the side of a mountain, over Sisyphus-sized boulders and across ice fields into thin air where my body hungered for oxygen. Every part of me ached.

Now I felt like I was suddenly cast into the centre of a scene in a sitcom. My first reaction was: what's that contraption for? I don't think anything can prepare you for the sight of an empty wheelchair, especially when it dawns on you that it's intended for your use. My initial response was to reject it. If I was going to get out of bed, I would roll over and stand on my own two feet. That shouldn't be so difficult, if I could only find both of my legs. And my right arm didn't appear to be functioning. That was a problem. It hurt. I could feel the pain, especially when it spasmed. I needed it to push myself up, but my arm appeared to be "on the blink."

What a curious expression, I thought.

I turned and looked to Pat for help. Nicole had vanished.

Nothing was working. Everything I took for granted was "out of order." I half expected to find a sign to that effect hanging on the end of my bed.

One of the women pushed back the curtain that separated me from my roommate. I wanted to see him, finally, to see what it was that caused him to have such a low self-image. To my surprise, he was gone. Sensing my alarm, Pat told me that while I was sleeping someone had come to take him to imaging.

Then I saw Nicole standing by the door. She seemed pleased with the little drama that was unfolding. I remembered that the three of us had just been settling in, talking about their evening and, quietly, oh so quietly, talking about the shenanigans and theories of my roommate, when these three had showed up. Why was Nicole obviously cheered by what she saw? Everything about the actions of the physiotherapists was at odds with the way I felt. They were so busy and assertive, while I was as docile as a herded animal.

With the curtains drawn back, the room looked expansive.

"Are you ready to try walking?" the man asked.

On the one hand, this seemed a very stupid question. Of course I wanted to walk. I wanted to pull on my jeans, shirt, socks and shoes and make a beeline for the exit. I wanted to spend the night tucked up in front of a fire with my family. I wanted Owen, my son, with us, with me. I wanted to feel like I'd felt the day before I'd had the stroke. Truthfully, I wanted my full brain back.

On the other hand, the blunt reality was that my body felt weighed down, like a tree branch bent low to the ground after a heavy snowfall, and my brain was in free fall, rapidly losing touch with thoughts and images that connected me to the familiar. How I longed to kick my way through a pile of leaves and stare up through the bony shapes of maple and alder trees at the winter sky.

Movement seemed a vain exercise, a promise of the impossible, the sort of promise we make to the dead, to always remember them in the moments before we begin to forget them. What a grim thought, but I had been thinking a lot about dying over the past few nights. Ghoulish thoughts, in images befitting a bad horror flick in which I was being buried or cremated alive. Someone had forgotten to take my pulse. Or to put a mirror up to my nostrils to check for breath. Did mistakes like this actually happen? Carelessness and indifference, I told myself, are habits of the living.

Naturally I wanted to try walking, but how?

I nodded, and I saw Nicole clap her hands. Since she clearly wanted this, I was determined I would do it, for her.

"Yes," I said. "Let's try walking." At least I think that's what I said.

They must have understood me, because with what seemed like one swift simple movement, they had me perched on the side of the bed with both feet placed on the floor in front of me. I wasn't at all sure how they had managed this manoeuvre, but there I was — seated upright. Then they wrapped something around my waist and put slippers on my feet.

"This is a transfer belt," one of the women explained. "It will help us to keep you balanced and give us something to grab onto in case you start to fall."

In case I start to fall. That was reassuring.

"We'll try to walk as far as the door, to Nicole, and one of us will come behind with the wheelchair in case you need to sit down. The other two will be on either side of you holding onto the belt and supporting you under your arms. Okay?"

Again I nodded.

Was this really happening? I glanced up at Nicole who, across the vast span of the room, urged me on. She was saying something like *Come on, Dad, you can do it*, but between worrying about failing her and the bemused idea that my three assistants viewed me as an oversized toddler just out of diapers, all I could think about was standing up. Then suddenly I was on my feet. I can't remember if they gave me any sort of warning before they hoisted me up, but immediately I noticed that my left leg was reasonably firm while my right leg seemed to be missing in action. I panicked and wanted to sit back down.

"It's okay," the male therapist said. "We've got you. You've done really well. That's the hardest part over with. Just take a few seconds to get used to the idea of standing."

So I stood, slightly stooped, looking across the room at Nicole. Earlier, when we were together alone, I had broken down, unable to hold back my tears. I wept, uncontrollably. She had kept repeating that I was going to be all right, that I could heal from this, but for whatever reason I would have none of it. Then, like now, I was frightened that I would fail, that perhaps my condition was permanent, that I would not survive at all. I did not want to die. My brain then could not grasp her belief in my recuperative powers; and now, I was struggling to appreciate the tenderness with which she was willing me to walk across the room.

So I walked, shuffling, my left foot lifting as if it knew what it was doing, my right foot dragging behind like a recalcitrant twin. A petulant sibling. Each step was not only a gigantic physical task but drew power from every brain cell I could muster to help with the infinite calculations that each step took. Why was walking, something I had done with ease most of my life, so difficult? Distance to Nicole and the door, remaining upright, movement, body parts (especially the increasing pain in my gut), the physiotherapists on each arm, the wheelchair behind me, Pat (who was encouraging me on, as she always had, her love ever-present) — all became a part of an equation so complex I almost lost heart halfway across the room. But, no, I refused to give in. Between Pat, Nicole and this little group of therapists — my jazzercise group — they made me believe that together anything was possible.

When I reached the door where Nicole was standing, I experienced a curious marriage of elation, frustration, pride and weariness. Why? Why was my response such a mix of different feelings?

I was pleased that Nicole was happy with my performance. She applauded. She seemed genuinely excited. Thrilled, even. About what exactly, I still wasn't sure.

"Oh, Dad," Nicole said, "you did it. I'm so proud of you."

Pat was more restrained.

I stood there, bent over, looking down at my bare, pale legs reaching to the floor from below the hem of the blue hospital gown. They looked detached. I knew that at best I had actually walked only a distance of twenty feet. Twenty feet at the most, I thought, perhaps less. So what was the big deal?

"Yes, well done, Mr. Smith," the three therapists echoed.

Why was this a feat to celebrate? I searched their faces for a sign that they might be teasing me; or for a signal that they were humouring Nicole. But I detected nothing, only three deadpan expressions, followed by encouraging smiles, meant, as far as I could see, to disclose nothing. Masks, they wore masks, I thought — they were play acting. Why were they congratulating me? I had achieved nothing.

Okay, I had made it across the room with considerable difficulty. If I had been in better shape, I could have crawled the distance more quickly. And now I felt drained of energy and wanted to clamber back into bed. Why couldn't I stride out as I did on the golf course or stroll along as I always had, whether through the backstreets of London or Rome or along tidal flats or a trail in the forest close to home? My whole being sagged. This was not an accomplishment of which to be proud, at least not in my view. There was a rashness to their hoopla.

"Well done, Dear, this is the beginning. These are the first steps to a full recovery," I heard Pat say from somewhere behind me.

What was everybody talking about? Words, exuberant words, filled the air and yet they made little sense to me. They were the sort of thing you said to a child who you were trying to convince to swallow a spoonful of cod-liver oil.

Then I fell back into the wheelchair and folded up like a rag doll.

I sat there and gazed out into the hallway, past the trolleys, past the nurses coming and going, past the damaged people shambling along the corridor, to a vision of myself long ago, a youthful figure, somewhat athletic and short-sighted. With a full and vigorous head of hair. I loved books and music, gardening and walking. And poetry, yes poetry, unencumbered by criticism and unnecessary explanation. I loved the purity, both the pain and the joy, of its celebration of life; I loved the mystery at the centre of its geography, its searching language.

Then it trickled into my brain that I'd had a stroke. Stroke, yes, a stroke. The word resonated even more. I wasn't supposed to be able to walk.

Somebody had mentioned "disabled" to me at some point, a tone of regret in their voice. There had been talk that I might be paralyzed on my right side. That appeared to be true, which explained the struggle I was having with an uncooperative, unwieldy body. I felt legless. My torso dodged one way when I wanted to go the other way. My bowels refused to work, in spite of the stool softeners. My speech continued to sound like I was speaking from under water. And both my right arm and leg knotted up with spasms until the pain was so intense that tears came to my eyes, pain that was so unbearable I thought my jaw would break with the strain.

I was still hungry.

On the bright side, though, I had just managed to walk, at least after a fashion. I had stood up and, with assistance, crossed the room, taking baby steps, all the way to the arms of my daughter.

I had walked, I told myself.

Hadn't I?

Then the therapists gathered round, and each in turn shook my left hand.

"Congratulations," they said, "we think you're ready for therapy, even at this early date. You have great support here." They glanced at Pat and Nicole. "And you seem pretty determined. That's good. Your determination will go a long way towards assisting you with recovery."

I felt Pat's and Nicole's hands on my shoulders and then, following the therapists' lead, we accompanied the three of them on a tour of the ward, Nicole pushing the wheelchair, Pat by my side, watching over me, making sure I understood that I would never be alone. Her presence like a quilt, warm and comforting. Through the acute ward.

What a small space to be crowded with so much suffering, I thought, with so many old faces, slack and perplexed.

I didn't let Pat or Nicole see my anguish.

Instead, I imagined eating an apple, not whole, but as a warm sauce over ice cream or peeled and cut up and baked in a fine, fluffy pastry crust, served with a slice of cheddar. A yellow transparent apple picked just as it turned colour, from a deep lime green to the pale shade of the moon. Not what they used to call an eating apple but a cooking apple. Slightly tart, with a sting in its tail. Not an apple you would feed to a horse but an apple whose juices lingered like the summer sun on your tongue during a fall rain or winter snow storm. An apple that held the reach of a climb when you had scuffed a bare knee against rough bark. An apple with a short ripening season, testing your will to live another year.

At that point back in bed, I think I slept. Briefly. And lightly. For I soon became aware that Pat and Nicole had stopped whispering and fidgeting and had bolted upright in their chairs as though sensing something important was about to happen. Blinking my eyes open, I saw a woman quietly entering the room. Was this the moment I had been waiting for? The woman carried a notebook and pen, and a bag which I was to learn contained saltine crackers, a spoon, a plastic container filled with apple sauce, a paper cup and a box of juice. She was the "Swallow Lady." I was sure.

She was not at all like the feathered creature my imagination had conjured up — someone round and diminutive, with shortish legs, and an impish nose, like a tiny beak. I think by this time I half expected the "Swallow Lady" to swoop into the room on a pair of wings, perch above the bed and start chirping out commands.

This woman — handsome, tall, even elegant, I thought, dressed in her low black pumps and calf-length skirt — was perhaps sixty, although she looked younger. It was her presence that spoke of her years, not her grey hair or glasses. Only someone who had worked at her career over many years, happily and confidently, could carry time so well. She had a calm about her that comes only with experience and maturity.

I liked her immediately, before she'd even uttered a word, before she'd performed the first of her swallow tests. I think I trusted her smile.

Finally she spoke, with a slight English accent. She introduced herself. If she mentioned her name, I don't recall, but she did make it clear that she was a speech therapist, not a rare bird. She was here to see if my stroke had caused any damage that would temporarily or, if worse came to worst, permanently affect my speech or ability to swallow.

In spite of my slightly mangled words, I was determined to prove that my going hungry for several days had been totally unnecessary. The hospital's caution was irrational. Unnecessary. Inhumane. Extreme. I was perfectly capable of eating anything they could pile on a plate.

"I still know how to swallow," I insisted, my mouth feeling dry and my tongue swollen as if I'd accidentally taken a bite out of it.

She sat serenely and watched me carefully with her pale blue eyes. She was someone who had made a habit of observing.

By now I had reached a tipping point. For the past few days, my mind had been humming with objections to this forced abstinence. I was so hungry I wasn't willing to engage in a debate on the subject of swallowing. After all, I had been swallowing food and drink my entire life. I knew swallowing. For someone to argue the point with me seemed absurd. I intended to make it clear that as far as I was concerned she was wasting her time.

Now that we sat face to face, I felt uneasy. Her self-assurance undermined the urgent wish I felt to assert something of myself. What did a swallow test entail? No one had told me. I tried to find fault with her. Maybe what I'd taken for stylish calm was just disguising prim fussiness, which I would be willing to overlook if I could get past her swallow test to a decent meal. Now, as my imagination spun into fantasy, I was making the ordeal personal. I had worked myself into a senseless anger and I wouldn't admit that this frustration was probably covering up my own fear of failure.

"After a stroke," she explained, watching me with a curiosity that told me the test had already begun, "the majority of patients find it very difficult to speak. And they find it doubly difficult to believe they can't swallow. Often both are temporary impairments, but in extreme cases either one can be permanent. I don't want to alarm you, but before we can let you eat or drink we need to be certain that you won't choke."

Before I could object, she took a deep breath, nodded, and said, as if by rote, "It's for your own good. Aspiration (taking something, usually fluid, into the lungs), for example, can frequently be a serious problem and lead to complications like pneumonia."

She sat back, crossed her legs and appeared to be waiting for an argument I was sure she'd heard countless times before. I disliked being that predictable.

As much as I wanted to argue my case, she spoke with a conviction and concern that was hard to refute. She made it clear that if I persisted in impulsive behaviour I could be in danger of doing something that was sheer madness, not to mention silly and stubborn. I got the distinct impression that she was not about to let me be reckless.

So I kept quiet.

This was more than I had bargained for. How many hours had I spent winding myself up for this meeting? Torturing myself. Rehearsing my argument. I looked around the room. My roommate must have been back in his bed because the curtains were pulled. Daylight filled the room so I assumed he was asleep, preparing himself to invade my night and dreams. I was already tiring. Everything else was in its place. Pat and Nicole glanced back and forth between me and each other, their eyes begging me to get on with it. I could see their impatience. I think they were as eager as I was to know what constituted a swallow test. I had a terrible gag reflex and I was concerned that the "Swallow Lady" might insert a gadget down my throat. Why, I wondered, was a speech therapist concerned with my ability to swallow? The relation between the two confused me.

"Are you ready for the tests?" she asked. "They're really quite simple."

"Yes," I said finally, not letting her know how wary I was, although I was sure she could detect my fear. I was ready to show the bird woman . . . the speech therapist . . . I was ready to show *her* that I could swallow.

To my surprise, she then leaned over the bed and placed the fingertips of each of her hands gently on either side of my throat. Pressing down lightly.

"Could you try swallowing for me, please?"

"That's it?" I stammered. "That's all you want me to do?"

"Yes," she said.

What could be easier, I thought, but when I tried to swallow my mouth was dry and my throat constricted. To my embarrassment, I couldn't swallow. I didn't know why but I felt my lips quiver and I wanted to cry. This was not the way things were supposed to go. I had expected to breeze through the tests. Defeat was not in the game plan.

Now I had what I could only describe as a lump in my throat. The harder I tried the more my throat tightened up.

"Try moistening your mouth," she said. "You need to relax."

I closed my eyes and managed to work up enough saliva to swallow. I was astonished by the effort it took. Nothing between my lips and my esophagus worked cooperatively. Then, in much the same way as a heron's long neck appears to move in stages when it swallows a flatfish, my chin pushed forward, my neck stretched, and I swallowed.

"Good," she said, "well done. Very good." She paused and looked at me to see if her reassurance was helping. "Everything appears to be working properly."

Then she scribbled in her notebook before reaching into her bag and pulling out a little package of crackers, the sort tucked beside a bowl of soup in a highway diner. She removed the plastic wrapper and passed one of them to my good hand.

"Now, I want you to try eating this cracker, but do it slowly. In little pieces."

Immediately I took a good-sized bite and just as quickly found it almost impossible to chew. My jaw didn't appear to be working. The piece of cracker stuck to my tongue and the roof of my mouth. Gagging, I managed to spit out the small chunk I'd bitten off.

"Nibble," she said. "Try nibbling. Tiny, tiny bits."

I couldn't believe it; I was being given a lesson on how to eat.

"Like a mouse, you mean?"

As I spoke I wondered how anyone could understand me.

"Yes, if the image helps. Like a mouse."

I felt like such a fool. How could I not swallow?

I did as she suggested and gnawed away at the edges of the cracker. I found when I licked the surface the salt stimulated my salivary glands and slowly crumbs made their way down my throat. Then I recalled that when these same crackers were served with soup I usually dipped them in the soup or crunched them up in my hand and sprinkled them on the surface of the soup. I would watch the bits sink as they soaked up the fluid. There had to be a clue in that memory. So I waited until each bit of cracker was softened in saliva and then swallowed. Still, if this was the best I could do, I didn't think there was much chance I would pass her test. I didn't see food of any sort in my immediate future.

I felt totally dejected. Life without food, without the simple taste of an olive or grapes or chocolate, would be absurdly incomplete.

"Good, now try this. But sip it slowly this time. Rushing your-self won't help."

She made more notes then poured a small amount of apple juice into a paper cup.

With the first sip I choked, but then I managed to drink it down in driblets, forcing myself to concentrate on each stage of swallow-ing and taking in no more than a teaspoonful at a time.

Next she presented me with a small dish of apple sauce, one of my favourite foods. I couldn't believe my luck.

For several seconds I sat there in bed and thought, if I can't eat this, there's no hope.

There are certain things we embrace or do, or gestures we make, which have a solemnity that gives them almost a ceremonial role in our lives. From early childhood, apple sauce had become a ritual food for me. And eating apple sauce had a ritual formality to it. Warm or cold, it had to be of a certain consistency. Transferring it from the spoon to my mouth, forming my lips around the cool metal of the spoon, required a particular movement as refined as a conductor's at the head of an orchestra. My lips would caress the spoon in the same way a baton caressed the music. And then I would let the apple sauce settle in my mouth and savour the moist pleasure of the exquisite combination of sweet and sour. I didn't dare tell the speech therapist what I was thinking, but I was buoyed by my secret.

Much to my delight and relief, each tiny spoonful glided down my throat with ease. The flavour and texture not quite what I was used to, but, all the same, the taste, the taste was wonderful.

The therapist smiled and seemed to take as much pleasure from my success as I had. Even so, I detected there was something else she felt I needed to learn.

"You've done really well," she said. "You'll be happy to hear you've passed the test. But before I go, I'd like you to try drinking a glass of water. Slowly," she reminded me. "Okay?"

I was elated. I had passed. At last I would be fed. If I'd been able to jump, I would have, but at that moment I once again felt exhausted and was content to luxuriate in the thought of food.

Dejected, elated, exhausted — my emotions swung from one extreme to another in the space of minutes.

"Yes," I said. I would drink some water: what could be easier?

The first mouthful went down the wrong pipe and I started choking violently, my shoulders and chest heaving, as if I'd spent too long under water. When Pat and Nicole rose to help me, the therapist motioned them back to their seats. For several minutes I continued to sputter and cough.

Unconcerned and confident I'd learned my lesson, the therapist watched me struggle to gulp in air.

"For the first few weeks," she said, rather too matter-of-factly for my liking, "all of your food will be minced or puréed. The thinner the liquid the more likely you are to choke. Obviously, as you've just learned, water is the thinnest food we ingest. You must try to eat and drink slowly and carefully. This is only one of the many things you're going to have to *relearn* how to do. Swallowing is not as routine or as fail-safe as you might have thought it was."

At that point, although I concede I might have been dreaming this, as she packed her bag and notebook, I thought I saw her wink at me.

What I did know for certain was this: another thing I had taken for granted all my life was suddenly a total mystery. An enigma. *Relearn* — the word would become a mantra of the therapist community. A physical movement I had always assumed was automatic had become an enormous challenge, requiring step-by-step, neuron-by-neuron, planning. I couldn't just stuff something in my "gob" and expect it to find its way to my stomach. I had never considered how complex the parts of the swallowing mechanism were: my mouth, tongue, teeth, palates, epiglottis, larynx, pharynx, esophagus, trachea, uvula, all working together in unison. What had been learned over a lifetime had been knocked out of commission with a single blow. A single "stroke."

In fact, it would take months for me to relearn how to swallow with confidence. I don't think a day passed when I didn't suffer a fit of coughing after something went down the wrong way. Usually water. At my first dental checkup after the stroke, in midsummer, my dentist told me he had two other stroke survivor patients who were unable to swallow and were now tube fed. I was very fortunate, he told me. Of this I have absolutely no doubt.

What I have come to learn is that after a stroke the brain and the body have a whole new set of propositions to consider and carry out. To map out. To make the necessary repairs, they must work in harmony, because restoring what has been damaged is a very complicated process.

For the second night in a row, when she got home, Pat wrote to family and friends recounting my day and the "expert" assessment she was given of my condition, which would later be revised to "semi-serious" when the extent of the physical damage I had suffered was fully known.

As far as I can see, an accurate evaluation of the harm done by a stroke is impossible to determine. No one has the crystal ball that will reveal what's happened inside a patient's brain. There are too many variables at work. The damage can be physical or cognitive or a wicked-and-devastating combination of both. One patient might regain physical controls and skills relatively quickly but be lost in a cerebral whirlpool, unable to speak, think or remember something they did seconds before. Their confusion or amnesia could last for months or years. Another patient might be unable to move and yet be capable of reconstructing complex thought processes including, as I was, distant memories. Full physical recovery, however, may never happen.

Add to the equation, the patient's emotional well-being and the care they are receiving — from everyone concerned but primarily the support they receive from family and friends — and a stroke becomes a very intricate event to assess. A stroke, essentially, is a formula for chaos, a chaos whose debris will scatter widely and weigh heavily on everyone it touches.

November 22, 2012

Hi All,

Today saw Ron much improved over yesterday. Much has also happened. He's been OK'd to move to the Rehab unit as soon as he can be processed. If that doesn't happen tomorrow, then it probably won't happen until after the weekend. His speech is much improved. He walked from his bed to the door (with wheelchair and 3 therapists at the ready), passed the swallow test and is allowed solid food. Nicole and I took him for a wheelchair promenade of the premises.

The doctor from the Rehab unit said that he might be said to have had a "mild" stroke but for the fact that he can't use his right arm and hand. Therefore, the doctor would have to classify him as having had a "medium" stroke. He also said that there is a 90 per cent chance that Ron will not have another stroke during the first year, and an 80 per cent chance that he will not have another stroke in the second year. These sound like good odds to me.

More good news: Owen is going to be able to come for two or three days around Dec. 1st and my brother, Bill, is going to "slide across the Strait" for a couple of days as well.

Nicole returns to Vancouver tomorrow. I started a new paragraph here, since I'm not certain this should go in the "More good news" category.

I would say the crisis is over and the recovery has begun.

Love to you all,
Pat

The next morning my favourite nurse woke me for breakfast — for my second solid meal in a week. The evening before, as a matter of principle and pride, I had picked away at a small plate of minced beef, two ice cream scoops of mashed potatoes, gravy, peas and a dish of canned peaches. And now, here was breakfast. All I could do was peck away at what stared up at me from my tray. Scrambled eggs, orange juice, jam, dry toast. What an irony. After all my complaining, I wasn't in the slightest bit hungry.

The thought of stuffing food down my gullet made me feel like a turkey being readied for Thanksgiving dinner. The pain in my gut was unbearable. Even when I curled up like a caterpillar, hoping to reduce the pain, the pain continued. A knot the size of a medicine ball seemed to be lodged in my stomach.

With each passing minute, the knot was cinched tighter.

Throughout the night I had wakened several times and buzzed the nurse for help. On a couple of occasions two of them had transferred me to a commode where I had sat doubled-up for at least a quarter of an hour in the dark, behind the privacy curtain, listening to my roommate talking about the American military in Iraq. In Afghanistan. In Pakistan. Why, I wondered, couldn't he keep his thoughts to himself?

I needed quiet in order to focus on what I was doing. With every "working" muscle in my body I strained, trying to force something through my system.

Eventually my moaning silenced him and he became surprisingly sympathetic. I was shocked to hear him plead with the nurses to help me.

The nurses tried giving me more stool softeners, by the handful it seemed, but nothing was moving. My system was on shutdown. I hadn't had a bowel movement in close to a week.

To say I was severely constipated would be an understatement. At another time in my life, anything to do with defecation would have been the essence of a schoolyard joke.

The fact is that in North America we are private and prudish about most things to do with our "toilet." We reinvent the Three Bears in a toilet paper commercial. Little pieces stick to their furry rear-ends. Cute. But why? Why do we make such a fuss and have so many theories about toilet training? We go out of our way to deny our animal nature. Perhaps this explains why on playgrounds toilet humour is always a big hit. Kids love to defy convention and giggle about the unmentionable. Perhaps it has something to do with our living in large part in a northern cold climate, in countries with chiefly puritanical origins. On my aunt's and uncle's farm, however, shit was as common as flies and a part of the daily workload for my cousins. Of all the people I knew growing up, their family was the most comfortable in their bodies.

Despite the farmyard, and despite our childhood daring, or what we take to be daring, we generally learn in Western society to draw curtains around our language and our bodies. As one grows older, our youthful braying gives way to silence. Pretence. Our bodies have no animal nature or animal function.

John Berger in his essay "A Load of Shit" in *Keeping a Rendezvous* addresses this separation from nature when he writes about the need to bury a year's worth of guests' shit after spring thaw. "Perhaps," he says, "the insouciance with which cows shit is part of their peacefulness, part of the patience which allows them to be thought of in many cultures as sacred."

I'm convinced that at least as many euphemisms circulate around our natural bodily functions as moons orbit a wobbly course around the heavenly body of Saturn.

Mum's the word.

But not the right word.

Constipation is.

For a stroke patient, constipation is a tricky business because it can be a side effect of medications or the result of serious physical damage. Or both. I think most stroke patients suffer from this side effect, but no one likes to talk about it. Patients are just handed a few more little red pills, medicinal candy, in the hope that nature will eventually take care of the problem.

On my first visit to Paris in the early 1960s, I went to a public washroom below ground off a busy intersection somewhere in the centre of the city. This was a new experience for me. Vancouver, where I'd grown up, was a relatively small, insular place in the 1940s and '50s. Apart from the one unattended, underground washroom at Victory Square, the city lacked clean public facilities, although I think I recall seeing a few pissoirs strategically placed around the downtown core. At some stage the city council shut them down because they were "unsightly" and "smelly."

In Paris, the bathroom attendant was a woman, which embarrassed and confused me. I wasn't prepared for a multi-sex washroom. But, defensively, I followed the lead of others, paid the fare of a few francs, went to a stall, which was doorless, quickly glanced around, cautiously lowered my pants, sat down and stared at the floor. When I finally dared to look up, a middle-aged woman sitting opposite me smiled and gave me a petite wave with her fingers. I waited, as if I were expecting an egg to hatch. Eventually she stood up, straightened her skirt and left, but before she did so she gave me a very coy look.

In Tangiers I remembered going into a public washroom and seeing a row of holes with two strategically placed, slightly raised footprints facing me on either side of each hole. I couldn't deal with this. North American to the core, I puckered up and raced back to my hotel.

And now here I was, on the morning I was to move to the rehab unit, and the pain was getting worse with each second. When the pain had reached an unbearable threshold, the young nurse of whom I was so fond suggested she give me an enema.

"I think it's high time," she said, "do you agree?"

"Yes," I answered, "flush me out. Blast away. Do something," I pleaded, "anything to get rid of this feeling that I'm going to explode. Or implode."

I have to confess, though, that I was utterly ignorant on the subject of enemas. It was merely a "word" I knew — with certain commonplace, and more often than not, crude and fetid associations. I'd never had an enema and I had only a vague idea of what to expect, although somewhere along the way I had been convinced that the experience would be unpleasant.

Such ideas are nurtured to save us, supposedly, from our profane selves.

By this time I had lost whatever modesty I'd had when I'd been checked into the hospital. In a peculiar way my body no longer felt like it belonged to me. I was an experiment waiting to happen, and relieving me of the mass, the dam of excrement clogging my system, was a priority. I would have done anything to relieve the cramps, the surging waves of pain and nausea that now seemed the sole function of my body.

Much to my surprise, whatever the nurse did was far less invasive than I had expected. But an hour or so after she had performed the procedure, nothing had changed. The enema had failed and, if possible, the pain was worse. It was a blinding pain, the sort of pain that forces you to clamp your eyes tight, as if doing so will somehow shut out the source of the torment. You see flashes of light behind your eyelids. I was beginning to understand why "shit" is an expletive in most cultures. I kept repeating the word, as verb, in the hope that repetition would induce the action.

Shortly after Pat arrived, a stretcher was delivered to move me from acute care to the rehab unit, and two nurses lifted me from the bed to the stretcher. I was still writhing in pain. I squirmed and strained. Angry and exasperated, I didn't care anymore where I "took care of business." Not only had I lost any sense of modesty, I'd lost all self-respect.

"There is one last thing I can do," the young nurse said as she approached me and stroked my arm, trying to relax me, "if you're willing to let me try."

"Anything," I slurred. "Please, just do something." I paused and turned my head so she could see the tears running from the corners of my eyes. "I'm not sure I can take much more of this."

"Okay, but what I have in mind is quite invasive, is very, well, personal."

"I don't care. Just do it."

"Just do it," my roommate said from the other side of the curtain.

Pat, who was standing off to the side, agreed and retreated to the hall.

"I don't want to get in the way," she said as she left, although I knew she couldn't bring herself to watch what we both assumed was going to be awkward and perhaps distressing.

Faith, I thought, faith was what I needed. I needed to put myself completely in this young woman's hands, as I would in Pat's. In this time and place there could be no secrets. Words like gentility and correctness and decency no longer mattered; they were no longer

necessary to obscure and protect my personal habits and prefer-
ences. This was no time to be shy. It was like opening the blinds at
night and turning on the lights.

"All right, then, what I'm going to do is go in and get it myself.
If that's okay with you? My poking around might cause some discomfort, but I think it will work."

"Do it," I said. "Please hurry."

While the nurse went off to get a bedpan, gloves and whatever
else was required to excavate my innards, I suddenly thought of the
joke that had circulated in the schoolyard sixty years earlier.

Did you hear about the constipated mathematician?

He worked it out with a pencil.

As the nurse probed away, this joke from my youth repeated itself
over and over, like a tape looping on continuous rewind.

Yet what astonished me then about this whole incident, and still
impresses me now and fills me with admiration for this young
nurse, was the ease with which she conducted the exercise. She
chatted away about the weather, about her family, about the nursing program she had completed only five months earlier, about her
dog, as if we were sitting down at afternoon tea. Never did she
panic or allow her voice to modulate. She carried on as if we were
old friends. I don't know if it was her presence of mind or if it was
the fact that she was so conscientious, but she made the act she was
performing natural and made me feel human again. She gave me
back a little bit of my dignity.

In that simple act was the tangibility of compassion.

After she left and Pat had returned to my side, Pat said it was the
largest stool she had ever seen. To be honest, I wasn't interested in
dimensions or an accounting. For the first time in several days my
gut didn't hurt. The old tiredness returned, grinding me down,
testing my will to start pushing back against the lethargy that settled into my bones. But already I looked forward to dinner, even if
it was going to be minced or puréed.

And a quiet, quiet room.

As the porters and nurses readied me for the trip to the rehab unit, they pushed me forward on the stretcher. When I looked up, I saw a massive bulk, like an immense carapace, lying on the adjacent bed. On the pillows at the head of the bed, rested a tiny head, out of all proportion with the body to which it was attached. Gregor Samsa, I thought. This was the first time I had actually seen him, this young man I had construed as a monster, as a night-figure of pain and fatigue. He wore glasses, a mustache and a smile.

"See," he said, "I look grotesque. I told you so. I can read it in your eyes."

There was no point in my denying what I saw.

"I'm sorry," I said.

"Don't apologize," he answered, "as soon as I'm out of here I'll come visit you in rehab."

"Do that," I mumbled, trying to sound upbeat, but when I saw him struggle to move, like a beached giant turtle, I felt terribly guilty. They would never drain off enough fluid. Somehow I knew this; and I knew that he knew this. All I wanted to do was weep.

He was so young.

SEVEN

The Wheelchair
and the Urinal

"Don't fight me," he said.

"I'm not," I said.

Once again I heard that strangely garbled voice.

"You are."

He held me in a modified bear hug, trying to transfer me from the stretcher to my new bed in the rehabilitation unit. Somehow he had managed to get me sitting upright on the edge of the stretcher, then by gaining purchase under my arms he got me standing on two very wobbly legs, at which point I grabbed him with my left arm and clung to him like a bear cub to its mother.

I was terrified. As soon as I was standing, my entire right side collapsed like an accordion. What was happening to me?

"Relax," he said. "You need to trust me. I know what I'm doing."

Trust. This was one of those words I would soon learn was critical to every phase of my recovery. Trust, and the need to be brave.

We stood there like a pair of ballroom dancers suspended in an embrace, each of us determined to go in a different direction.

"Trust me," he repeated. "I've done this many times before."

Pat, my constant companion, the one who listened to me talk about my fears, who agonized over my every jolt of pain, who sat by patiently as I burst into uncontrollable fits of weeping, who listened attentively to my incoherent babble, who laughed at my jokes (because there were moments that were maniacally funny), who constantly reassured me that I was going to get better, watched on. I knew she wanted to help, but equally she refused to interfere. I admired her steadfastness, her courage.

When you lose something you have always taken for granted, trust takes flight.

The more he and I struggled, the more I tried to help. I wanted to show him I could still do something for myself, but my body wasn't responding to messages from my brain.

"You're making this very difficult," he said.

His green uniform smelled of cigarette smoke.

I knew that smell from when I had been a smoker.

Then I said to myself, "must trust," and I sagged into his arms. In one swift effortless motion he picked me up, turned me and landed me gently on my back on the bed, as if I were as light as a breath of air.

"There, that wasn't so bad was it?" he said, triumphant and slightly winded.

"No," I admitted, glancing up at him from the bed.

I felt embarrassed. Why had I doubted him? This was his job.

I had to admit I was impressed. Mike, my first contact with a nurse on the ward, was in his fifties, had an untidy mop of grey hair and a full, dull-grey beard. Not exactly the nurse I had expected. Slender and wiry, he looked more like someone you would meet on the docks or in a logging camp or slinging beer. He couldn't have weighed more than one hundred and fifty to sixty pounds and yet he had lifted and shifted me like a stuffed doll. The index finger on his right hand and the lower edge of his mustache were yellow with nicotine, not exactly an advertisement for the healthy life. Later, after I made some sarcastic comment about black lungs, he told me he jogged every day to work off the ills of smoking. It's definitely a bad habit he went on to admit, and I'm addicted. Stupid. I'm a nurse for God's sake. A health professional. And then he chortled, as if to acknowledge his awareness of this little irony.

"This is your wardrobe," he said gesturing at a piece of furniture that stood next to the bed. Then his shoulders slumped and he bent slightly at the waist. How had this tall, scrawny figure managed to transfer me from the stretcher to where I was lying? As I looked up at him, I was feeling more and more detached from the world around me. The room. The people. The bed. The unfamiliar sounds. The disappearing light.

Who and what had I become?

God, I thought, I'm helpless. And hopeless.

This was not what I wanted to be.

Scratching the top of his head, Mike recited a list I could tell he had repeated dozens of times before. "You can hang a few things. Dressing gown, a couple of shirts, pants — preferably with an elasticized middle that you can pull on without too much effort — and there's a drawer for underwear and socks. You'll be expected to get up and get dressed every day. We'll help you at first but an OT, occupational therapist, will be around in the next few days to show you how to help yourself. You can use these shelves," he tapped them with his left hand, "for personal items. Books, shaving kit and so forth. You're not by the window, but you have a sink in the corner here. No one else uses it. That's a bonus."

He paused and stroked his beard, as if this helped him form a mental picture of what he would say next.

Why was the sink a "bonus"? I couldn't possibly shave with my left hand, not unless I planned to audition for the role of Scarface, and the sink was eight to ten feet away to my right, the length of a footbridge over a local creek, and I couldn't even sit up on my own, let alone stand and walk the distance.

What if I fell in? I could drown after a snow melt or during the rush of spring runoff. I was daydreaming again, my thoughts free-wheeling. Birds trilled in the surrounding trees and underbrush, which grew along the bank of the creek, in amongst the salal, brambles and Oregon grape.

"There's the toilet, on the other side of that door," he pointed to the opposite corner of the room. "Call us when you need to go." He handed me my buzzer. "Just press the button. And don't leave any valuables lying around. In fact, it's best if your missus," he nodded at Pat, "takes home everything of value. Anyone can walk through the ward and you won't always be here. For good stretches of the day you'll be in the gym working with a PT, physiotherapist."

Just then another nurse entered the room with an empty wheelchair, black with sleek and shiny chrome spokes, frame and handrims.

When I squinted I could read her name tag. Alison.

"This wheelchair is yours," Mike said. "It belongs on the ward so don't let anyone else borrow it. Wheelchairs have a habit of disappearing around here. Alison has taped your name on the back, so look at it as your responsibility to safeguard."

Why was I its guardian? And if someone did decide to purloin it, what was I supposed to do? Yell "stop," and if they didn't, chase after them with my curses? "Hey asshole, I'm the cripple here." At least that I could do as the thief retreated into the distance, although he or she probably wouldn't understand a word I said.

"Mine?" I asked, and I looked at Pat.

Just when I thought shifting rooms and floors was a sign that I might be the beneficiary of a miracle, her look of acceptance suggested she might be seeing some permanence to this contraption.

The wheelchair was an omen. Good or bad, I wasn't sure. Either way, it confirmed that I was truly paralyzed on my right side. Up until this very moment I had continued to hold out hope that whatever was causing the continual pain in every limb of my body would soon disappear and that my lack of mobility was temporary. I continued to view my condition as a nightmare in which I was a reluctant participant. I was still convinced that I was going to wake up, climb out of bed, walk to the car and drive home.

As hard as I tried, I couldn't wrap my brain around the idea that I was destined to spend my days in a wheelchair. It didn't make any sense. Fragility is common to all of us but, with a combination of good fortune — being born in the right place at the right time — and comparatively healthy habits, it rarely becomes an issue in our lives; and, when one sees oneself as a strong and confident person, frailty of any sort is impossible to imagine.

At sixty-nine, I was still a relatively young man. Admittedly, in my youth I had played rugby and had taken a few good knocks to my head, but all the same . . .

"You're lucky," Mike said, "this bed's been empty for a couple of nights. Waiting for you, it seems. Somebody up there must like you. Getting to therapy from the fourth floor as quickly as you have is unusual and could be very beneficial."

He paused, as if suddenly doubting his prognosis. "We'll see," he added.

He pulled the curtain along its track, and for the first time I could see the rest of the room, which was fairly large by hospital standards, and my new roommates. Three of them. All men. From their posture and hair colour, I guessed they were all older than me. But there was no logic to this assumption. What remaining hair I had was silver and when they caught a glimpse of me, they'd think me a bit of an old billy goat.

The two men closest to the window were curled up on their sides, backs to me, apparently looking out at the last of the light draining from a low, cloudy sky. Dull and threatening. The third man, directly opposite me, slept sitting up under the glare of a reading light above his bed. Every so often he would mutter a few incomprehensible words, then snort and his lips would shudder with a snore.

"I go off shift in a few minutes," Mike said as he inched towards the door. "Is there anything else I can help you with?"

I shook my head.

Where had the day gone? Time had begun to tilt, as if it travelled on an elliptical orbit in the same way Earth did. Some moments had interminable duration, while others flashed by like photographs. Brief and theoretical.

Leave us, please, I thought, trying to send my wish to Mike. Telepathically. I wanted to be alone with Pat for a few minutes before she packed up. Each time she departed now, her absence left a hole that became harder to fill. And fathom. My connection to the world was becoming increasingly tenuous, and her presence — looking into her eyes — helped to reaffirm my sense of belonging.

I remembered once a baby crow attempting its first flight from its nest in a cypress tree in front of our house on the beach. Instead of taking flight it had toppled from branch to branch to branch to the ground where it huddled confused and at the mercy of any hungry cat or raccoon passing by. We had placed it on top of a towel in a shoebox. It had stared up at us with the largest pair of blue eyes. A few hours later, with encouragement from its parents, it had flown back to its nest. From then on, over the years, it lived in the trees around our property and followed us wherever we worked in the garden. Always cawing, as if we shared a common language. Connections, no matter how nebulous the links, are vital to who we think we are.

Soon it would be dark and, by the way Pat was beginning to fret, I knew she wanted to be on her way. Several hours spent traipsing around after me, helping me interpret and cope with each new little problem — problems which under normal circumstances would have been infinitesimal but for me now seemed insurmountable — had to be mind-numbing. When I glanced at her face she looked haggard — with black circles under her eyes and sunken cheeks — yet invincible. Her will to continue was everlasting. Her strength was one of the things I loved most about her. She was not going to let this "event" defeat us. Trample us under.

Us, I repeated. Us.

No matter what I sometimes felt or thought, I was not alone. I had never been alone. The stroke had happened to both of us. As bewildered as I felt, I needed to keep that notion in mind. Even when words no longer made any sense, my separation from the world was not as great as I frequently imagined. And though I still had to work out to what extent this was true, I knew that my recovery would be a fight we would both share.

"This is much better than upstairs," she said, "much roomier."

"Yes," I agreed, my voice still sounding strangled, rising from some strange doubting place in the depths of my body. "Much."

As difficult as it was, I tried to keep any hint of disappointment out of my voice. I didn't want her to know I dreaded her departure.

She sat on the edge of the bed. She was whispering, an expectancy in her hazel eyes that suggested I should be grateful.

"And quieter. You must be pleased with that?"

"Yes," I blurted out, but without the slightest conviction.

Where was my old bouncy self? Could she tell I was faking it?

I was a prisoner, both of my body and the bed. What could possibly be satisfying about that? I lay there motionless. Again I wanted to weep.

"Look" she said, directing her gaze towards the window where the orange glow from street lights had just flickered on. "During the day you'll be able to see out the window. Listen to me," she said, "you have to insist they keep the curtains pulled open. Being on the ground floor is a plus. And overlooking the parking lot's not so bad. You'll be able to watch people come and go. And the road across the way is where I park the car. You'll be able to see me arrive in the mornings. This way you'll be able to keep in touch with the outside world."

She hesitated, perhaps detecting that I was not as comforted by these words as she had hoped.

"Sort of," she added.

In touch! With what? I was tempted to ask her as she stood up and gathered her things. She squeezed my hand and kissed me.

What must it be like, I wondered, to kiss flesh that had lost its meaning? I could still feel her touch — other survivors, months later, would tell me that at the time of their strokes they had lost all sensation in their skin — but *my* skin felt like it had separated from who I was. I had the strange sensation that Pat wasn't kissing me. Or that she was kissing an older version of who I was. Someone I no longer recognized.

As I watched her leave, I began a descent. To where I wasn't sure. No sooner had she packed her things, than I missed her. Before me, all I could see was a darkness opening up that resembled a bottomless pit. A void. An absence of something. Of everything. The sort of darkness, I imagined, that formed at the heart of a black hole.

Around me, all I could hear were songs of emptiness.

What had happened? Had I fallen asleep? My mind twisted and turned, as if trapped in a maze. Fog enveloped everything. And everything moved in slow motion.

Before Pat had left she had told me that tomorrow she would return with her brother, Bill, in tow. I was pleased about that. It would be good to see him. He was always jolly, a man of the theatre, with a flair for the subtle nuances of the absurd, especially those that leapt from the bizarre or unexpected corners of our daily lives. He acted and directed, although I had always suspected that his first choice was to climb into someone else's skin for a few hours. I still chuckled when I thought of him in his role as Sgt. Binns in the TV series,

The Beachcombers. Or as Poe in the tense and tone-perfect voice of his one-man-show based on "The Raven."

His presence, his laughter, rooted deep in his belly, would lift my spirits, I was sure of that.

Even so, as soon as Pat departed, the sense of loneliness and disconnectedness returned. How to describe that place, those feelings of despair?

So much negativity.

First and foremost, I was still afraid I was going to die. This feeling haunted me for weeks, especially when I woke in the wee hours of the morning to the hushed silence and eerie, artificial twilight of the ward. The stroke encapsulated my world. Took over. Then, after dwelling on all the things I hadn't said or written, especially to Pat, Nicole and Owen, I would tell myself, "*Nothing is ever completed, we live in a state of anticipation,*" and I would cry myself back to sleep.

So much uncertainty accompanied stroke prognosis, and even though Pat repeated Dr. Jill Bolte Taylor's insistent and wise supplication from *My Stroke of Insight,* "expect full recovery," I couldn't get enough reassurance. I wanted to be forgiven, but I couldn't think why. I hadn't done anything wrong that I could recall. I wanted to apologize for failing to live up to other's expectations. But whose? And again, why? Was it guilt? If so, why was I feeling guilty? Nothing made sense. When I exhaled, it was a struggle to draw another breath. Perhaps the place I was attempting to describe was the place of grief we came to know after a loved one has died. A hollow place: hard and cruel and lonely.

Or was it simply an indulgence, a case of despair craving despair?

Shortly after Pat left, we had been served dinner, a sombre affair which for me included puréed meat, vegetables and a fruit. As promised by the "Swallow Lady." In contrast to what I'd experienced on the fourth floor, my new roommates let me sleep, uninterrupted, for a couple of hours. What a treat. If I knew nothing else, I knew I needed rest. My brain repeated the word "sleep" as if it were an invocation.

The two men who occupied the beds by the window were amputees. One was deaf, with a mouth frozen in a smile, and the other was angry, at everything as far as I could see and hear. He was miserable, his phantom limb still haunting him. He curled up in a ball, clutched his bedding and whimpered. The man opposite me, Jack was his name I later learned, watched me from a distance I couldn't begin to comprehend. His eyes seemed light-years away. Every so often he nodded and smiled at me as if we had just been introduced in one of the gardens at Versailles or on one of the moons of Jupiter. He was somewhere else, definitely not here.

Next, the nurse who had recently arrived for the night shift came to take our vitals — blood pressure, blood sugars, pulse — a ritual they continued to repeat four times a day over the following weeks. Was the heart really that fickle? These tests were supplemented by the woman who came every other day from the lab. I watched anxiously as she inserted a needle into my arm and withdrew several test tubes of blood. I flashed back to the chemistry set I'd had as a kid and the experiments I conducted in the attic of my parents' house. My father, by this time in his life an accountant, was a patient man, but with the first explosion and the accompanying stench, my junior lab was shut down for fear that the house — the house he had built with his own hands at the end of the Depression — would be burned to the ground. Why were they taking these samples, I wondered? What could blood possibly tell them about my paralysis or about the mess my brain seemed to be in?

The nurse's final act before the lights were dimmed was to give us our medications. In those early days, as I've said, I think I must have been on at least a dozen different drugs. At least one for depression, a couple for blood pressure, one for loosening stools, some for lowering cholesterol and blood sugars, others for muscle spasms and pain. The spasms were the worst. Without warning, the muscles in my right leg and arm would suddenly contract and an excruciating pain would shoot down each limb. I wanted to scream but instead I would grind my teeth and my fingernails would dig into my hand, leaving red welts where I had almost broken the skin. My entire right side seemed to go into involuntary cramps as if someone were tying me up in little knots. Or stretching me on a rack. Both limbs would vibrate with the strain. Yet pain and cramping were the two conditions on which the drugs seemed to have little or no effect.

These contractions would continue for months. As would the pain.

Even today, two years later, the spasms recur, almost daily, although the pain has lessened. I also burp and sneeze involuntarily, as if the stroke gods think I need one final reminder of their power over free will.

Just before she exited the room, this new nurse turned and asked if I would like a portable urinal. I looked at her blankly. I was more than twice her age and I had no idea what she was talking about. I knew what a urinal was but "portable" made no sense.

"To pee in during the night," she explained, as if I were a child. "Then you won't have to call us every time you need to go."

I could understand why that would be a benefit to everyone concerned, but I couldn't transfer the image I had of a porcelain urinal attached to a wall to something portable.

"I'll fetch one and you decide," she said.

A few minutes later she returned with an aqua-coloured plastic container about the size of a quart of milk, its neck bent at a forty-five-degree angle four or five inches from the tapered end. It came with a handle and a three-inch opening at the top. I looked at it in dismay and with total bewilderment. How? How did it work?

She explained that I'd have to sit up, which I couldn't do, or roll onto my right side towards the edge of the mattress and position myself so that I could stick my penis in the opening. Held at the correct angle, she told me, it would be like pissing in a bottle.

"No problem," she said.

Maybe not for you, I thought, but since dinner I had been thinking about how alien my body felt. My corporeal being seemed to belong to another world. After dinner I had tried to roll onto my right side, but nothing worked. Besides, the pain was intolerable. And I could no longer shift onto my left side because I didn't know how. My left arm and leg moved, but I'd lost the operator's manual.

"Try grabbing the bed rail with your left hand and pulling yourself over, onto your right side," the nurse said. "Like this," she said as she placed my left hand on the railing.

I remember looking at her with puzzled misgiving, but I did what she said.

Such a simple suggestion, such a simple gesture as placing my hand on the railing, had huge ramifications. The proverbial light bulb went off in my brain. What I hadn't been able to figure out on my own suddenly made sense. With my hand placed on the railing, it dawned on me that I could use it to help roll onto my right side. The nurse didn't tell me how to pull myself over; she left me to work out the mechanics on my own.

In such a simple act, in the bringing together of two images, like a tree felled to build a bridge over a huge chasm, lies the origin of metaphor and the solution to, and understanding of, so many of our problems. The brain's power to make connections, to invent or envision solutions in a time of need or desperation, is astonishing.

Much to my amazement I managed to roll over, but I felt fatigued. And I hurt. I had done so little and yet I was physically and mentally weary.

"Try giving it a trial run," she said. "Hold the bottle by the handle in your left hand and just make sure the bottom of the bottle is tilted down. You'll be fine."

As I teetered on the edge of the mattress, I peed into the bottle, without a thought for the nurse who stood by watching me.

I gave a big sigh of relief.

There is a fine line between constructive advice and advice that frustrates and humiliates — the sort of advice that makes you feel as thick as a fence post and slightly less than human.

I was elated. I had actually managed to do something on my own.

"When you're finished, just stand the bottle on your night table. Then we'll know when to empty it."

She smiled.

"Well done," she added as she shuffled out of the room.

I could have kissed her.

In the weeks and months that followed, this little teal-coloured bottle, which reminded me of the sea, would become for me a major symbol of my recovery.

Diagonally across from me, in the bed by the window, the smiling amputee watched television. My other two roommates were asleep.

Covered by a single sheet, I lay on the bed and stared at the ceiling which was constructed with acoustic tiles filled with holes, the sort of tiles that were supposed to deaden sound. I began to count the holes, but I would get only so far before my mind strayed to thoughts of what might-have-been or my eyes wavered and I lost track of the row I was counting.

At dinner I had tried to eat with my left hand, spilling half the meal onto the bedding or onto my nightgown. I was definitely not ambidextrous. When the lights went out and all that was left was a moonlit glow from the hallway, I just lay on my bed and drifted down, and then down again, into an abyss.

Without memories occupying my brain and reminding me of who I was; without my old roommate talking up his latest conspiracy theories and challenging me with his cockamamie ideas; without newscasts, newspapers, magazines, radio, TV reminding me of the strange-but-familiar antics of the day-to-day world; without books, paintings and music speaking their urgent and controversial languages about space, time and different ways of seeing; without a sense of continuity between what I had once been and what I now seemed to be; without Pat, I was lost. Adrift. "Without" appeared to be the extent of my vocabulary and was becoming my story.

Or perhaps it was the opposite. After Pat had left, maybe I simply had too much time to think. I had not suffered a massive stroke, such as the stroke that had torpedoed and quashed Jean-Dominique Bauby, but I had had a serious stroke, one that had disabled half of my body and had left my brain scrambling between stasis and chaos. The old adage "he doesn't know if he's coming or going" suited me perfectly. At certain moments I felt like I had arrived at a still point in time, while on other occasions my mind seemed to spin out of control.

Perhaps, I thought, I felt this way because for the first time I was fully conscious of the fact that I was disabled. That I was paralyzed. And disconnected, in a way that I didn't yet quite understand. I was no longer me. In an uncomfortable way, I was beginning to feel sorry for myself.

When you have a stroke it is difficult if not impossible to believe that this pummelling is happening to you. Even though your body feels bruised from the pain, even though you have seized up like an old gearbox, if you are still capable of thinking, nothing computes.

I was devastated. The more I looked around the room, the less I seemed a part of it. My surroundings were more like a stage set, something temporary, and the length of the production uncertain. Would tonight close out the run, I wondered?

Would I die?

For years now I had subscribed to the theories that described the Gaia principle. Our interconnectedness with the planet — animal, vegetable, mineral. For as long as I could remember I had embraced the idea that Bill Bryson had recently advanced in his *A Short History of Nearly Everything*:

> Every living thing is an elaboration on a single original plan.
> As humans we are mere increments — each of us is a musty
> archive of adjustments, adaptations, modifications, and prov-

idential tinkerings stretching back 3.8 billion years. Remarkably, we are even quite closely related to fruit and vegetables. About half the chemical functions that take place in a banana are fundamentally the same as the chemical functions that take place in you.

It cannot be said too often: all life is one. That is, and I suspect will forever prove to be, the most profound true statement there is. (415)

On the other hand, I worried that perhaps my separation had been going on for some time and the stroke had simply accelerated the process. I no longer appeared to belong to the pool of energy to which I assumed we were all connected, and that I was convinced was the consciousness of the universe.

I now felt as though I were living inside something akin to a canning jar. There was no escape. I was trapped.

Voices and ideas came from everywhere. I couldn't stop them. In the normal world you can choose to tune things out. You can take a break from the mayhem that characterizes our daily lives. You can decide what you want to hear or think. I had lost that skill. My defence mechanisms were no longer working and, without them, I worried about my sanity.

I became obsessed with how to connect. I was asking myself, "How do your seemingly random thoughts — your internal narratives and fragmentary memories such as your sweeps through Europe — serve as a way back to who you still are? Or are you randomly wandering through a parallel universe in which you either begin to reclaim an old identity or frame a new one? And how many dimensions are there?"

While a part of my brain was damaged, other parts seemed to be working overtime to compensate for what I had lost. Memories, I was convinced, were the one touchstone I shared with my old self. They worked like a metaphor to help heal the separation and establish my claim on "being."

Most significantly, I began to realize, I'd forgotten how to forget, a normal function of a healthy brain. Inside the stroke, inside the jar, I felt as though I could hear all the voices that had ever spoken in what was an unending record of reality and the imaginary. And I had no idea where they converged and separated. In this sense, reality for me was always at one remove. Eternity always one step behind itself.

My first night on the new ward, alone with these thoughts, was terrifying.

Throughout the night I wept.

I drifted in and out of sleep into the early hours of the morning. A couple of times I buzzed for help and was shifted by two nurses to my wheelchair and then wheeled to the toilet where I sat until I rang for them to do the same in reverse. After my earlier bout with constipation and after taking so many stool softeners, I feared that I might be incontinent. Shitting the bed would be the final humiliation.

I occupied a place that was so remote it might have been prehistoric, with only the vaguest hint of any connection to who I was or who I might have been in a past life. I wondered if I was genetically connected to anyone or anything on the planet.

My thoughts cycled round and round on an unforgiving memory circuit until Pat arrived with Bill just before lunch. I could hear Bill's booming voice the moment they stepped onto the ward. As he walked through the door, his tall, bearded figure brought comfort. A cap was perched jauntily to one side of his head. Perhaps because they were brother and sister, I knew instinctively he would provide Pat with some relief from me, from her interminable vigil. The tension, not to mention the monotony of it all, had to be exhausting. How was it humanly possible for her to continue? How did she keep her spirits up? My grief flowed, unrelenting, and my condition was grotesque if not repellent.

Their arrival was a welcome break from Jack who had spent most of his waking hours since breakfast staring at me from across the room. What was his story? At times I got the impression that he thought he knew me, his lips almost forming a greeting; at other times, usually when he drooled, I felt like a specimen, pinned for study on a lepidopterist's board. His eyes stared through and past me, took flight through time zones and across galaxies.

Jack.

Jack, who had shouted out "bird" several times during the night, who had startled me awake with this word that he pronounced as verb, noun, question, plea and command, had undergone a very severe stroke. On top of his dementia, the nurse told me. He was not in very good shape. The nurses referred to him as the "Bird Man" because he called them "Bird" or inserted "Bird" randomly into conversations on any subject. I stared back at him, a little more discreetly, I hoped, than the way he had been staring at me. What was happening behind those eyes, so vacant, so forlorn? Was this what I could expect from my stroke? Would I reach a point where my brain would collapse in on itself like a piece of rotten fruit? Like a rhododendron blossom wilting at the end of its short life?

I remembered a quote from the Buddha: "O monks, work out your liberation with diligence, decay is inherent in all component things."

This message suddenly had a certain urgency to it.

Pat and I had arrived late on the ward the previous afternoon and in a bit of a panic before the weekend officially started — a time, we were warned, when inertia slowed care down to a crawl. Nurses had been heading off shift, a new crew arriving. Everything had felt unsettled. Pat had rushed off without seeing much of my new lodgings. Now she proposed the three of us — her, Bill, me — take a tour of the facility. She asked Alison, who had returned to duty that morning, if she could help Bill and her move me into my wheelchair. Alison pointed to an instruction written on the whiteboard above my bed indicating that no fewer than two nurses had to be present for me to make such a "transfer." The instructions

were illustrated with stick figures as if for a primary-school class. I
grew impatient. Why couldn't Bill and Pat help? They were strong,
healthy individuals, quite capable of lifting and throwing me about.
Once again I felt like I was being held hostage to a condition for
which I was totally blameless. Why did everything have to be so
bureaucratic? Such a production?

In retrospect, Alison, who I liked a lot for her blunt honesty, was
just doing her job and doing what she thought best for me, but the
procedure of shifting me from the bed to the wheelchair was nerve-
racking. I felt like I was the special project of some mid-level military minion in logistics who was making sure I was offered a safe
ride to the front line. As cannon fodder. So we waited as Alison
fetched help and I was safely transferred.

Hunched in my wheelchair, I glanced furtively into each room
we passed as Bill pushed me down the corridor to the main nursing
station — operation central, an island of computers, fax machines,
phones and endless printouts — then on to the lounge.

The lounge was an all-purpose room in which I would later take
mirror therapy. It was also the room in which patients were encouraged to gather for lunch around several large tables pushed together
in the centre of the room. Someone had decided that it was good for
residents of the ward to mix and mingle — I could see the memo:
FRATERNIZATION IS THERAPEUTIC — but everywhere I
looked I saw gloom, overarching gloom. So many patients appeared
to have given up. Few left their rooms, and when one or two occasionally strayed out it was as if they dragged a sledge of stone behind them. Lassitude had won out over active reclamation. This
malaise was infectious and was something I wanted to avoid.

Our wing, set aside from the rest of the hospital, next to the psychiatric ward, was reserved for amputees and stroke survivors. (*In
my experience and from what I've read, stroke survivors are often shunted
aside, because no one knows quite what to do with them. Brain "insult" is
still a huge medical mystery.*) This annex of the complex was not a

happy place, although God knows what I expected. No one who had survived a stroke was going to be dancing on her or his bed or doing back flips and somersaults. There was no reason for celebration. Survival beat the alternative but had its own load of misery: the gradual and inevitable breakdown of body and brain, as far as I could see. These people were damaged souls, some more than others. Everyone had been shocked into disbelief. Everything drooped, like the unhappy jowls of a bloodhound.

When we're ill we tend to dwell on the darker side of the colour palette, we drift in amongst the greys, purples, midnight blues and blacks, rather than gamboling through the rich and warm shades of begonias — yellow, red, pink and orange.

But thankfully, Pat wouldn't let me pine away. Sulking was forbidden. Doom and gloom out of the question. She was not going to let me feel sorry for myself. Suck it up, I could hear her say, as we cruised towards the gym, which was locked up for the weekend, but held the promise in the weeks and months to come of my standing on my own two feet and reaching with all my strength for the summit of Everest.

Her optimism was unsentimental, her love urgent and visceral. We had arrived at a point where all illusions had been swept aside and a blunt, in-your-face reality stared us down. Gunslingers in a deserted and dusty Tombstone street. In her heart, she knew we were going to win this fight; it was that simple.

Nor were most staff tolerant of any signs of bowing out. Of quitting. Of allowing patients to plunge into some distant evening afterglow. How the nurses remained so upbeat was a mystery to me, because between patients moaning and groaning and family members bitching about the state of health care in general, and care for their loved one in particular, they were besieged by ingratitude.

The feisty wife of one of the amputees in my room, a wizened and arthritic woman in her eighties, a woman who clearly loved her husband dearly, found fault with everything the nurses did. What she didn't know from past experience, from decades of nurturing and caring for her own family, she had looked up on the Internet and was happy to show these youngsters how to do it.

"He's in pain all the time," she said. "It shouldn't be like that. You need to do something. Not just give him another pill."

Her tongue clucked as she adjusted his pillows and stroked his brow. She made a point of showing that their relationship was special. Probably they had been together for over fifty years and by now his bones were her bones.

She was tireless. On and on she went with her complaints. The dressing on her husband's stump was either too loose or too tight. The ointments were wrong. In the old days, she would say, this is how we would have done it.

The nurses, in turn, had the patience of Mother Teresa. And the tenacity of bulldogs.

As I travelled through the halls in my wheelchair in the weeks to come, what I heard was a chorus of voices raised in a song to healing. Rarely did I hear anger or frustration or annoyance escape a nurse's lips.

Back at the room I dozed between wakeful moments of conversation. We must have talked about something in particular — family, travel, Bill's summer place on Pender Island which he was always repairing — but if so I have no recollection of what it was we discussed. Eventually Pat and Bill left, dinner was served, and I slept on. Jack yelled out "Bird" and I rang for the nurse. Either he couldn't find or couldn't reach his buzzer. Between blinking eyelashes I watched two nurses adjust his oxygen mask, pillows and the tubing that ran in and out of him. He smiled and moved his lips. "Thank you." I was pretty sure that was what he said as I hovered in the dreamy realm between joy and fear. I was happy to be alive but still terrified because no one could tell me precisely what had happened to my brain or the entire right side of my body. The words "*You've had a stroke*" continued to swirl in my mind. Why couldn't anyone be more explicit?

"A broken brain," they said, "is not like a broken leg."

"Nor, for that matter, a broken heart," I mumbled.

The two amputees complained about the sores around their wounds, where the leg had been removed from the knee down. Both men stared at the absence as if belief would grow them a new limb. I wondered which was worse, losing a limb or losing your marbles.

Neither, I decided.

Or both.

Comparisons didn't help. I wasn't ready to sort out the paradox.

Sometime in mid-morning the next day, Bill returned alone to the hospital, as we'd agreed, just in time to run off to purchase two coffees. It was difficult for me to imagine going through an entire day without Pat. Without seeing or hearing her. Yes, there had been times when we had spent time apart, on occasion for several weeks, but this was different. It wasn't so much my missing her that worried me as the thought that I might never see her again.

A close friend of mine from England had lost his wife in a car crash. He had returned home to Wiltshire from London to the harrowing news of her death only a few minutes earlier on one of the older highways. A narrow, twisting road that runs from Swindon to Marlborough through some of the most beautiful countryside in the UK. A head-on collision on a dangerous stretch of road. Needless to say he was gutted. The last he saw of his wife was in hospital when he went to identify the body. No one can be prepared for the suddenness of such a tragedy. No words exchanged. No hug or kiss. No endearments. No preparation, if that's at all possible. Mourning, I had thought, would always feel incomplete.

As I sucked lukewarm coffee through a straw, Bill told me that Pat had said that, with her free time, she was going to catch up on housework. He had insisted she get some rest, but we both knew the minute he stepped out the door she would be putting the house back in order. Seeking normality. No one is prepared for the role of caregiver. The demands. The time dedicated to a singular and daunting purpose. There are no courses or instructional manuals on the subject that speak in anything but generalities and platitudes.

The particulars of care are learned on the fly, especially the need for stern love and blunt honesty. Perhaps it's something maternal, something that springs from a feeling of solidarity. Being there, offering support and love for a stroke survivor is a caregiver's most precious gift. I knew Pat was exhausted from her constant presence by my side, but I also knew she wouldn't heed Bill's advice. She had standards and they needed to be upheld. She would put a record on the stereo or a CD in the player, probably Leonard Cohen, and settle into a familiar routine. Quite possibly singing "The Future" or "Hallelujah," thoughtlessly, out of habit.

Over the next few hours Bill told me about his latest plans. He was writing a film script, a mystery-romance built around genetic modification. The idea was bizarre, totally bizarre, but I loved the madness of it — and his enthusiasm. It wasn't at all clear to me where he was going with the idea, but it seemed the sort of thing that could and likely would easily morph into comedy. He was also helping a friend with his script, a science fiction thriller that tested all the boundaries and conventions of the genre. They were looking for funding for script development — they had a producer for the project and Bill had already spent considerable energy finding actors and scouting out locations — but money, there was the rub. Finding enough cash was always the biggest hurdle to making a film.

He continued, breathlessly, recounting the plot, developing the characters (at least as far as he had conceived them), setting a scene, speaking the dialogue, describing costumes, filling in the backstory, all delivered like a happy lunatic. Bill delighted in slapstick. Where would he insert the banana peel?

At certain moments he had to pause while I caught needed rest. When I blinked my eyes open, he carried on without missing a beat. It was a wonderful monologue about theatre and film, about love and the cosmos, filled with endless details about the stars, earthly and heavenly, in which my silence converged with his exuberance. As he perched on his chair beside the bed, I watched his hands inscribe the space between us, between the inert and bustling worlds, as if he were a master conductor connecting the two. I waited on his every word.

In short, he made me feel as if I was included in his world.

There are several things I learned from Bill's visit. I realized how much I needed to be loved and how much I needed to love back. I also needed the empathy of friends and family, and, even more importantly, for them to treat me as they always had. I wanted to feel human again. I wanted to feel as though I belonged. Ordinary sympathy, by contrast, actually hurt. When I sensed people were attempting to be kind and considerate — that they were walking on eggshells — when I felt that their message was guarded, I withdrew into the stroke. Such messages reminded me of how fragile I was, reminded me of how close to death I had come.

Some things can't be prettied up.

I knew that I was different now, that I scared people, that I reminded them of their own mortality. This self-pity was a weakness we all shared and was now something I wanted to avoid. Seize the moment, I thought, and its eternity.

Friends who had come to visit me so far were affable and tender, and most stayed only for a short time. This was a relief and a blessing. As I lay in bed, fatigue joined hands with pain and I slipped happily into a listless torpor, as if I were a creature accustomed to bedding down for a long hibernation. In my dreams, in an attempt to reassert a sense of self, I traversed the streets and byways of memories I thought I had long ago forgotten. Streets filled with the clutter of a fulfilled life: thousands of books, records, photographs, paintings, pottery, golf clubs, my father's shop tools, my mother's china, clothes that no longer fit, shoes I never wore, old clocks that hadn't ticked or tocked in years, an old Leeds United scarf, porcelain figurines, old furniture, especially an old rocking chair my grandfather had made. All this and a loving marriage that had survived for forty-five years. And two remarkable adult kids.

I couldn't wait to see Owen.

Was it Sunday or Monday? I don't recall. As the new week got underway, I luckily vaulted to the top of the list for a weekly shower. This was my introduction to the inner workings of the stroke ward. Much to the annoyance of my roommates, my arrival on the ward corresponded to the beginning of a new weekly shower rotation. Up until now all I had received was the occasional sponge bath and those usually hastily performed. To put it bluntly, I smelled. The two amputees were furious and made their displeasure known. I had arrived latest on the ward and should be last. "What the hell's going on?" I heard them complaining. Happily for me, no one paid them any heed. I happened to be in Bed #1.

First thing in the morning, two nurses came to the room and transferred me to a commode. Before my admission into hospital, I had never seen such an apparatus — essentially a toilet on wheels. A removable bedpan sat below the toilet seat. The benefit of this new throne was that it was made of chromed metal, plastic and vinyl. It could be pushed into the shower without fear of water damage.

I was readied for the excursion. All I wore was a green hospital gown, tied loosely at the back. My private parts dangled below the seat, a breeze rushing past them. A volunteer, a woman in her forties, homely but charming, pushed me down the very public hallway, past nurses and other patients beginning their day, to the shower room. By this time I had lost all sense of modesty. Proprieties of any sort had disappeared from my thinking and were to be completely washed down the drain over the next quarter of an hour.

I can't begin to tell you how good this felt, being scrubbed down with a washcloth and soap from head to toe, and then showered off. For a brief spell I forgot that I couldn't move half my body and that a complete stranger was being openly intimate with every nook and cranny of my physical being. We talked without need for explanation and laughed. For a moment I was miles away from my troubles.

A year later, a friend of mine who had suffered a serious stroke ten years earlier, and to whom I'd gone for advice about recovery, told me about his first shower. Basil is Irish and the volunteer who had assisted him had recently emigrated from Ireland. During the shower she noticed he had a rather large umbilical hernia.

"I call that my *dickeydo*," he said when she pointed it out.

"Your what?" she asked. "I've never heard of such a thing."

"My *dickeydo*," he repeated.

She looked at him quizzically.

"Yes," he smiled, "because it sticks out farther than my dickey-do."

"Oh," she said, "I wouldn't let that bother you; you're still a handsome fella."

He told me that at the time he had felt extremely grateful for this little exchange, for this interlude of normalcy. It announced his refusal to give in to what his stroke threatened to steal from him. His humanity, yes, but perhaps more importantly, his sense of humour.

EIGHT

Jack the Bird Man

What is a stroke? This question still befuddled me.

Technically I understood the mechanics of a stroke but its implications were much broader than how a clot or bleed assault the brain. There was more to it than a coagulated mass being driven from the heart to an artery in the brain — in the same way that an earthquake is more than tectonic plates shifting somewhere along a fault line off the coast beneath the ocean floor. An earthquake is equally the tsunami that follows or the nuclear reactor knocked off-line and leaking radioactivity into the ocean; or homes destroyed and lives and livelihoods lost; or a way of life swept out to sea, possessions carried across an ocean and, years later, washed up on beaches a continent away. Similarly, a stroke is paralysis; loss of identity; loss of cognitive skills, speech, hearing, swallowing; loss of family, friends, livelihood; a loss of home and mobility; a stroke is equally a loss of the love that sustains us all.

Over the next several months of rigorous therapy, as both an in-patient and out-patient, I was to formulate an increasingly complex, confused and contradictory understanding of what a stroke entailed. I soon discovered that most patients were as baffled by the "bombing" of their brains as I was. A few doctors shook their heads and admitted to a limited knowledge regarding anything to do with the brain. Others nodded their heads and referred to computer images they felt told the story, alluding to dark masses recently formed in the frontal lobe, Wernicke's area, the cerebellum, the sensory cortex, the occipital lobe, Broca's area or brain stem, for example, as if they were tornado or hurricane sightings on a weather map. From sources as varied as informed definitions provided by medical professionals to anecdotal accounts spoken and written by actual stroke survivors, I developed a widely expansive and distressingly divergent awareness of this word that had changed my life.

I knew a stroke was sometimes referred to as an "insult to the brain" or as a "brain attack," two metaphors that were certainly apt, but that were also far too general to be useful as anything other than a general description of the event itself. Neither described the fallout from the calamity or even hinted at the long-suffering and painfully slow road to partial or full recovery. Neither explained what was going on inside my head. Nor did they tell me why my whole body had seized up and was knotted with continuous pain. But I was still optimistic.

What my stroke came to mean for me personally when I began my years of therapy was much more subjective. Much more primordial and intuitive. Much more a matter of loss on a massive scale — identity, voice, muscle mass, body control, independence, movement, belonging, self-esteem, emotional control, brain function, recognition and so on. I was suddenly plagued by depression, fatigue, spasticity, paralysis, and a mind that freewheeled with none of the safety nets or regulators that people are accustomed to having at their beck and call in their day-to-day lives.

The filters that normally protected my brain by weeding out unwanted or unneeded information and experience no longer worked. My senses, especially sight and sound, were on high alert, receptive to the slightest stimulation. My startle reflex, for example, was so keen I was continually jumping "out of my skin" at the smallest movement or the quietest whisper. I soon realized that regaining my defence systems was going to require the same concentration and patience as relearning how to walk, talk and think.

I was like an infant.

I'm convinced that a large part of "growing up" is learning how to filter out the extraneous from our daily lives. Perhaps this explains youthful rebellion. What, I wonder, accounts for our growing conservatism as we age?

During my first week in rehab, my sister-in-law, Barb Osaka, by profession a hospice nurse of close to forty years, presented Pat with a copy of Jill Bolte Taylor's *My Stroke of Insight*.

"This book will help," Barb told Pat.

And it did — it helped Pat to understand what I was going through, physically, and to a degree, emotionally — in spite of the fact that Taylor and I had suffered different types of strokes — hers hemorrhagic, mine ischemic — strokes that appeared to have decidedly different outcomes. At that time, I was still unable to read Taylor's book, mostly because I couldn't hold an object of any sort in my right hand, and I had the concentration of a brick.

A few months later, when I was finally able to lift a book in my left hand and flip pages with the same hand by cornering the book against some other object, I was grateful for Taylor's thorough and insightful explanation of the anatomy of a stroke.

And yet, even so, as the survivor of an ischemic stroke, I felt I had a contrasting story to tell.

Taylor writes about her stroke: "Within four brief hours, through the eyes of a curious brain anatomist (neuroanatomist), I watched my mind completely deteriorate in its ability to process information.

By the end of that morning, I could not walk, talk, read, write, or recall any of my life."

My stroke, by comparison, was much more gradual. After a few hours, however, I, too, was unable to walk, move my right arm, my speech was impaired, and I was unable to write, although I think I would have been able to read had I been able to hold a book or concentrate long enough without hungering for sleep. But, unlike Dr. Taylor, at no stage did I lose my ability to process information or recall my life. Certainly I was confused and bewildered; and in all likelihood my mental processing was a bit irrational. Some things made perfectly good sense, others did not.

So many of my experiences seemed totally different from hers. For example, she regained physical control relatively quickly while my right side was badly damaged, and a year and a half later was still behaving like a defiant and rebellious child. My forearm, wrist and fingers refused to bend in the same way they had pre-stroke. Spasticity had taken over. And whatever part of my brain coordinated my sense of balance with my legs and eyes was still out of commission. On the other hand, I never lost control of my cognitive abilities, as she claimed to have done. Yes, I was withdrawn and scared, but I still knew what was going on around me. I was quite capable of problem solving.

Up to a point.

Early Monday morning, eight days into my stroke, I had my first encounter with an occupational therapist. She was a thin, sinewy young woman, blonde and pale, quite attractive, who I felt was far too shy and timid for the job she had been assigned. When she started to talk to me about my "condition" she smiled, but her face flushed. Why was she embarrassed? She made notes in a binder in the largest cursive script I'd ever seen. It was more like drawing than writing. I remember being fascinated by the way she held her pen, by the way she squeezed it in the "V" between her thumb and index finger and not with the tips of her fingers. She questioned me about my goals — now that I had suffered a stroke.

"What do you hope to be able to do for yourself?" she asked.

"I don't know," I answered. "I've never had a stroke before."

My voice still sounded as if I were speaking from inside a bucket. How could she possibly understand me? All my life, language had been one of my main passions and strengths. The day before my stroke I had been editing a poetry manuscript, courting the muses for inspiration. Now I mumbled incoherently like a chattering magpie.

I sat in my wheelchair and glared at her. Her question seemed to me careless. I'd lost half of my body, I no longer felt like I belonged to the human race, my brain kept taking tours into my distant past, and I was exhausted. Rather than answer what seemed to me absurd questions, I wanted to crawl back into bed and bury my head under a pillow. I was beginning to think that the questions people now asked me originated in a fragile "other" world. They came wrapped up like fine china with "handle with care" labels attached and surrounded by an aura of pity.

And yet I worried that I was being totally unreasonable, unfair and perhaps a little insensitive. I knew she wanted to help me, and she was determined to do so with poise and attentiveness, something I didn't feel I deserved. In particular, she wanted to show me how to help myself; she wanted to show me how I could put on my socks, pants and shirt with the use of only one hand. When she tried to guide me through the simple steps to put on my shirt, I got tangled up trying to push my head through an arm hole and my right arm was dead weight nowhere to be found. I panicked. I felt like I was a contortionist trussed up in a straitjacket, and when I realized I couldn't move I feared I was going to be suffocated inside my own shirt.

Like a cartoon character, I tried to punch my way out.

My second attempt went no better. Trying to put on clothes was like entering a maze. Soon I was tied up, body parts going in all the wrong directions. I felt like an insect trapped in a spider's web.

After she got me unravelled, she showed me different ways to brush my teeth and wash up with only one hand — with my left hand, an appendage which until now I had rarely used for serious tasks. It was completely useless. I tried to run a face cloth over my head and around my neck without poking out an eye. It had never occurred to me before now how dependent I was on my right hand. The occupational therapist's show of concern seemed pointless to me. I was totally hopeless. I lacked any of my old hubris.

And yet, and yet Laura (I think her name was Laura) was tireless with her encouragement. She was helping me to see that I could relearn the basics.

Outside, a few rays of sunlight broke through a cloudy sky, splashing faint golden light on the far corner of the room. Pat was dropping Bill off at the ferry that would take him back to the mainland, and she would be late arriving. Waiting was becoming a new habit for which I was developing patience.

In mid-morning I was told by one of the nurses that I had an appointment in the gym with one of the two physiotherapists who would be working with me over the next few weeks.

"Do you know your way to the gym?"

"Yes."

"Then you'd best be on your way. Your appointment's for ten."

It was then I realized they expected me to wheel myself to the gym, a distance of about one hundred and fifty metres. Good luck, I thought. I couldn't begin to go in a straight line. The minute I pushed or pulled on the one wheel I could grip with my "good" left hand, I did doughnuts. My right arm hung lifeless, resting in my lap.

"Drag your left foot backwards along the ground at the same time as you push, and keep your right foot on the footrest," a nurse told me.

When I tried to do what she suggested I made it a few metres before I veered right and smashed into the wall.

"The effort you make now will pay dividends in the future," she added, her words sounding like an advertisement for an investment company. "Perseverance," she said over her shoulder as she tended to Jack, "that's what it takes."

I repeated this lurching motion several times, scribing little semicircles before once again smashing into the wall, until I passed through the double doors into one of the main corridors running through the hospital. Now I was stranded and alone. Then I looked down the hall to the right to the sign outside the gym. One hundred metres left to go. It might as well have been on the other side of the world, several lifetimes away. Thinking I might hitch a push, I tried to look plaintively into the eyes of everyone who passed by, on their way to an appointment or on their way to meet someone for coffee or off to perform surgery, but no one noticed me, at least not consciously. At waist height, I was beneath their radar. Besides, for most people I was just another familiar part of what they expected to see in a hospital hallway. For some, though, perhaps for those who were just visiting, I was an obstacle to avoid, possibly infectious, definitely out of order, and they gave me a wide berth.

As I sat in my wheelchair in the middle of the hallway and watched the pedestrian traffic surge around me, like water around a rock, I began to think of all those people passing me as the "temporarily enabled." While I knew this sounded terribly bitter and resentful, I was searching for some way to explain my having recently become "permanently disabled." The suddenness of it all still percolated in my brain. What had happened to me could happen to any one of them, to all these perfectly "enabled" bodies rushing past me, and it could happen to them just as suddenly.

Without warning.

Were they aware of this?

I took another run at manoeuvring the wheelchair down the hall, but again I swerved to my right and almost collided with an elderly woman who was trying to slip past me. She was towing a basket of what smelled like freshly baked bread and rolls. She was in a hurry, puffing a bit and anxious, perhaps using the hospital as a short-cut home.

At the rate I was going I would arrive at the gym just in time to turn around and repeat the journey back to my room for lunch. This lesson in self-motivation seemed to me utterly futile.

Then, to my surprise, I bolted forward and sped quickly, in a straight line, towards the gym.

"I'm assuming we're going to the gym," I heard Pat say from behind me.

"Yes," I said, trying to pivot my head. "Is that you? Of course it's you. Yes, thank you," I sputtered, my tongue tripping over itself, over an odd mixture of nagging frustration and gratitude. "I'm already late. They expect too much of me. I'm supposed to wheel this bloody contraption all the way down this hallway with one hand. I keep smashing into the wall. I'm a hazard out here, for Christ's sake, to myself and to others."

"I know, I was watching. I think they want you to do as much as you possibly can for yourself. They say it's good for your morale."

"Not if I *can't* do it," I slurred. "Repeatedly running into a wall isn't good for anything except a case of bruised knees. Failure is one thing, I can accept that, but you can't teach a stone to swim. My time would be better spent on doing therapy that makes what they want me to do at least feasible. I'll know when I'm ready to go solo. And happily do so, crashes and all, but until that time I could use a little help, thank you very much."

As we entered the gym a young woman approached us. Her face was covered in freckles and her dark hair, not quite jet black, was done up in a ponytail. When she grinned every muscle in her face warned "impish." Watch out now, her smile said, I have a trick or two up my sleeve. I could easily imagine her as Annie in the musical *Annie Get Your Gun* based on Annie Oakley's life. Then I wondered, where had that image come from? I hadn't been to see a musical since the fifties when my parents took me to Theatre Under the Stars in Stanley Park in Vancouver. Those had been magical nights when song soared amongst the gigantic fir, hemlock and cedar, and rose into the darkening starlit sky above the amphitheatre.

"Hi, I'm Deena, one of your physiotherapists. You'll also be working with Vicky. We're known to our patients as the *physio terrorists*." Then she laughed at her own small joke, laughter as clear as the tinkling of wind chimes. "But don't be alarmed. We're really quite harmless."

I fancied her the second I noticed the unexpected play of light in her brown eyes. And the smile, dimples and all, which came to her face as naturally as breathing. Anyone, I thought, doing a job week in and week out caring for people who had recently had a limb cut off or treating people whose brains had been whacked and who were physically and mentally damaged, often to the point of being mute or vacant, had to be quite special. And to be filled with so much enthusiasm and joy was extraordinary.

What a miserable and gruelling parade of misfits we were, lumbering about in our mental fogs.

Over the next hour she slowly introduced me to the equipment spread around the gym. She told me what I could safely use. Initially I could try my hand (a curious turn of phrase considering the circumstances) at the stationary bike and the weights on pulleys. That was it! But first we would be working on simply getting me to a standing position. Our main goal was to build up enough strength in my legs so I could make the transfer to my wheelchair unassisted. I needed to reconnect my body to my brain, perhaps forge new pathways between the two.

"Two things," Deena said. "Always remember to apply the brakes when you go to leave your chair. It's a matter of safety. Otherwise you could end up on your fanny. Or break a hip. And repetition," she continued, "repetition whether with light, light weights or with repeated movement is the key. That's what retrains the brain. And builds up muscle memory."

"Will I recover?" I murmured.

"We'll see. All in good time." She paused. "Typically, recovery is slow, very slow, after a stroke. You need to be patient."

For the next month, my physiotherapy would be filled with a lifetime of frustrating and embarrassing failures, usually when I was attempting to perform tasks I would have been able to do in my sleep in my former life. Everyday things, things I had done for decades on automatic pilot, like button my shirt, tie my shoelaces, zip up my coat, buckle my belt, brush my own hair and teeth, feed myself, things I took for granted, not least of which was going to the bathroom on my own — *everything* became an insurmountable obstacle and a test of my will.

Over the first few days in rehab I noticed many changes to my emotional and spiritual being as well as to my body. I could feel the changes to my right hand, which in my imagination now looked like a crab pincer. Try as I might, I couldn't even lift it to confirm my suspicions. And I could feel my right foot turn inwards with each spasm, like the feet of kids struck with polio in my youth. Would I now scuttle sideways when and if I recovered movement? Would I carry this stigma around with me as they had? Only at that moment did I realize how callous and tactless our responses had been to the deformities this disease had caused. Drop foot, braces, a shrunken limb. But what shocked and surprised me most was my gradual descent into what can only be described as an abyss. An absence. Looking around me I saw a mood of hopelessness. I was being sucked down as if into quicksand. It was suffocating.

"Every stroke is different, every stroke is unique," the medical and therapy staff kept saying as if each of them had been programmed with a recorded message. I was puzzled by these often-repeated phrases, because the treatments seemed to be essentially the same. For everyone. And most treatments addressed physical damage, not cognitive loss. Brain damage didn't seem to be on the menu for recovery. Dead was not a euphemism. Dead was truly dead, as far as the stroke-damaged brain was concerned.

Like robots we all wheeled ourselves into the gym and climbed aboard a piece of equipment, rolled around on a mat or bench, walked with the assistance of a walker or between parallel bars, and, for the more adventuresome, climbed and descended a low set of stairs. One day, Deena asked me to kick a soccer ball. As I staggered to catch my balance, I knew immediately that athletics of any sort had likely vanished from my future.

I saw patients abandoned, either because they couldn't perform the physical rehab or because they had simply given up. It was easy to become discouraged. To withdraw or want to hide. When you saw others struggling to stand up or roll over, you were looking in a mirror. And then, I wondered, how could they treat something that was supposed to be unique — something as distinctive as a fingerprint — how could they treat that oneness, that singularity, with the same potion or the same set of drills? It simply didn't make sense.

Here's the point.

Everyone could see the physical damage *I'd* suffered and they clearly had some idea of how best to deal with it, but no one appeared to be the least bit interested in my mental state of being. No one asked what my thoughts were or where they led. No one questioned me about the landscape and atmosphere of the stroke world. No one wanted to know its secrets. Where was their inquisitiveness? I think they actually believed I was still a part of their world, as crippled and as marginalized as I was. When my body felt pain or if I had a headache I was given yet another pill. But no one knew what was going on in my brain or in any other patient's brain for that matter, and everyone involved in therapy seemed resigned to watching each of us scramble to find a mental footing.

It was universally acknowledged that depression was a serious and inevitable side effect of stroke. I could certainly vouch for that. And from what I had observed, so could all the other stroke patients.

Naturally, therapists tended to respond to their successes, and because they were unable to get inside the brains of their patients they used physical results as their measuring stick. I could understand why this was the case, but I wondered whether or not a key to resolving some of stroke patient mobility problems resided in understanding the cognitive damage each of us had suffered.

Maybe, just maybe, understanding and explaining the extent of damage to the patient's brain would make work on the mats, therapy stairs and trampoline easier and meet with greater success.

My bouts of melancholy continued. Initially I had been buoyed by the constant attention from Pat, relatives and friends. Now Pat, who had been present every day, felt I was comfortable enough for her to take a little time away from me for herself. Perhaps a full day, with any luck. Presumably the drugs I was taking provided me with protection against a sudden lapse into serious depression. But as the safety nets broke down and the barrage of doubts and losses increased, the drugs seemed less effective. My emotional roller-coaster ride accelerated.

I was a participant in an emotional circus.

My spirits rose and fell, as if I were riding a merry-go-round. Some of the ride was due to the medications, but most was the result of mood swings. I felt I no longer belonged in the world. I had been banished to live inside a stroke with a disabled mind. At night, after the lights were turned out and the nurses had made their final rounds, my mind tossed and turned and spun, as if trapped in a cyclotron. That's when I felt most adrift, in a small boat on an angry sea. That's when I plunged into the darkest recesses of my mind. Vertigo overcame me. Lifelines had gone. Nothing made sense. All signs of life as I knew it had disappeared. Time dragged. It had all the weightiness of prison time, at least as I imagined life in a small windowless, concrete cell.

I couldn't stop myself from crying. I was being sucked into a whirlpool that had all the worst and insistent hallmarks of a soap opera.

My initial nights on the rehab ward were a nightmare. I would lie in bed and listen to my roommates' moans, a grisly sound that rose from some faraway place, perhaps from the bottom of some icy crevasse. Every so often Jack would yell out "Bird" and I would feel his frustration.

One bad scene piled on top of another.

"What's wrong, Jack?" a nurse asked from behind her flashlight.

"Bird," Jack said, not a question, not a statement, but a plea.

Then the nurse, fiddling, adjusted his pillows and blankets.

"Bird, bird," he said, his brow furrowing, his voice crusty.

"I don't know what you mean," she said. "You need to help me."

"Bird," he pleaded again.

And then she adjusted what I assumed was a catheter or his oxygen mask and he closed his eyes. I watched him settle, uneasily, to reclaim whatever dream sustained him.

On the morning Owen arrived I decided I'd had enough. For two or three days I had been lingering in the depths of a dark hole I had dug for myself. This moping would not do. Was unacceptable. I remember waking up at six and asking the nurse on duty to help me out of bed. I wanted whoever was on duty to make a point of doing this every morning, before the others were even awake. I wanted to be sitting in my wheelchair by no later than seven. And I wanted to be taken off the anti-depressant medication.

That'll be for the doctor to decide, I was told. He's the one who'll have to make that decision.

"No," I said, slumped in my wheelchair, "no, that is what I have decided."

Patient's rights, I would insist, like Perry Mason. Or Ironsides from his wheelchair, both roles played by Raymond Burr who went to school with my adoptive mother in New Westminster.

ight or wrong, I had concluded that the combination
ıs taking contributed to this downward spiral I was ex-
They made me feel dopey and listless, a little like I
imag͟ı͟ slug or snail felt as they slithered from one lettuce head
to another. And in addition to removing me from the anti-depressant medication, I was going to insist they take me off the drug I
had been prescribed for spasms. I could endure the pain when my
leg and arm went into sudden paroxysms, but the spasm drug itself
left me feeling as though I had been squashed. As soon as I took the
little white pill I was sure I was losing "me." My brain retreated into
a gloomy soup and my body felt like it was pixelating.

Now, with the clarity brought on by a new day and with the decision to take at least some responsibility for my own recovery, I
began the practice of staring at and concentrating on my right hand
and arm. What I wanted to achieve was mindfulness and visualiza-
tion. My goal was to travel throughout my body with my brain,
starting with my arm. If I devoted some of my free time every day
to meditating on and generating positive thoughts towards a certain
part of my body, I was convinced I could aid the healing process. I
certainly had nothing to lose with the idea.

For the past two days, after lunch, I had been doing a half-hour
of what was called "mirror therapy." My initial reaction to this activity was one of skepticism. A woman who wore what I remembered being called a pageboy haircut and who conducted the sessions as if we were a kindergarten class began each one with the
same spiel: "We are about to fool your brains." As I looked around
the multi-purpose room at the other patients, I was tempted to suggest to her that it wasn't going to be much of a challenge. On the
other hand, everyone was attentive, especially Scottie and Marie.
Perhaps I was wrong and we all clung, no matter how grim our
prospects, to hope, the sort of hope that accompanies the purchase
of a lottery ticket.

Promises, promises, I thought. Often the indeterminate moment
is defined by the promises we make to ourselves.

In mirror therapy, a mirror about fifteen inches high and twenty-four inches long is set in a wooden stand and placed on a table in front of each patient. The mirror is angled out at about thirty degrees from the patient's traumatized shoulder. It is important that the damaged arm and hand be hidden. As with any magical trick there has to be an element of the unknown.

In my case the therapist placed my right arm and hand behind the mirror. Then with my good hand — my left hand — I performed several simple exercises in front of the mirror, which I stared at with as much intent and concentration as I could muster. At first I pretended I was watching a puppet show, but soon, once I had decided I wanted to believe, I sat on the edge of my wheelchair, and stared fixedly in the mirror as hard as I could. And blanked my mind. No thoughts now, I told myself.

I drummed the fingertips of my left hand on the tabletop; rolled my clenched fist at the wrist; flipped my hand over and back from palm up to palm down; formed a fist and then flexed my fingers; rolled my flattened hand, fingers down, onto its side and back. I did this slowly, so my brain was taking in the movement. I tried extending each finger from a closed position and then reversed the movement. I did each exercise for about two minutes followed by a brief pause. And then repeated the set of exercises for between twenty minutes to half an hour in total. I stared into the mirror unblinkingly. I knew that registering the movement in my brain was critical. You couldn't let your mind or eyes wander, as some of the patients did.

"Remember, the goal of these exercises is to fool your brain," said the therapist in a monotonous tone. She stood, limp as an old cardigan, beside the upright piano someone had donated to rehab and that no one played.

What I saw, of course, was a reversed image. I thought I was looking at my right hand doing the movements. Not my left hand. My brain had been fooled.

Or had it? I wasn't sure. My right hand and arm still lay on the table behind the mirror like a lump of potter's clay, ready to be worked.

I thought of this repeated movement in the mirror as another form of meditation. While some patients found the repetition either boring or exhausting, I decided to view it as something that might benefit me. I was prepared to accept the therapist's claim that I was tricking my brain into believing that my damaged hand was making the movements.

I was determined to embrace this little deception.

In retrospect, rather than fooling my mind, I think these exercises helped to forge new pathways between the hemispheres of my brain. I took the routine seriously and twice a day wheeled to the room with the mirrors and did the exercises on my own.

One day, after a few weeks had passed, Nicole was visiting. She was sitting opposite me when she suddenly jumped to her feet and shouted that my damaged hand had mimicked the movement of my good hand. I didn't believe her. I'd felt nothing. When the therapist walked in and confirmed what Nicole was saying, I let out a whoop, lifted my paralyzed arm, and much to my amazement, flung it in a circle, hitting the mirror, which went sliding across the table and almost landed in Marie's lap.

Poor Marie. She smiled at me and tears rolled down her cheeks. I could tell she was pleased for me. Marie, who spoke only French and who must have felt doubly isolated, inside her language as well as inside her stroke, had become a comrade. We encouraged each other, whether in front of the mirrors or in the gym.

"*Bon, bon,*" Pat would tell her during the exercise. "*Tu as fait du bon travail.*"

I had movement in my arm for the first time since the day of my stroke.

"*Incroyable!*" Maria sobbed and shook her head.

By using mirror therapy in combination with my new form of early morning meditation — where I sat in my wheelchair and focused on my hand and attempted to travel in my brain down my arm to the tips of my fingers — I was hopeful that I might recover partial if not the full use of every part of my body. Soon I was telling anyone who would listen that I had travelled to the pads at the ends of my fingers.

"I'm there now," I would say.

"How did you get there?" they would ask, humouring me.

"I don't know," I stammered. "Perhaps along my damaged nerve paths or . . . or . . . perhaps down paths of longing, I don't know. All I can tell you is that I'm inside my fingers."

The energy of my entire body seemed to be concentrated in my fingertips.

When I started this meditation practice all I could see was the surface of my arm and hand, the skin with hair growing out of it, freckles, blemishes, moles, wrinkles around my wrist, pores and nails, especially the half moons at the base of each nail, but with time and focus I was beneath the surface where I could feel the flow of energy that ran through my body. Perhaps it was an awareness that travels on one's pulse. But I was there, that was all that mattered. Through meditation.

My "thinking and spiritual being" was in my fingers.

It was a beautiful sensation because it gave me hope.

Later, when I reread Hemingway's *The Old Man and the Sea*, this meditation I had performed reminded me of Santiago. When the old man hooks into the largest and most magnificent fish he has ever seen, he speaks to the different parts of his body, not as though they are detached or separate from him in some way but because they are so much a part of him and his actions. They have an immediate connection to his narrative. He expects his hands to behave as they have learned to behave. From habit, ritual, nature. There is no separation between mind and body. He needs concentration, kinship and a sense of wholeness to land the giant marlin, in the greatest contest of wills in his long life as a fisherman.

My right hand can hold it as long as it is braced, he thought. If it relaxes in sleep my left hand will wake me as the line goes out. It is hard on the right hand. But he is used to punishment. Even if I sleep twenty minutes or half an hour it is good. He lay forward cramping himself against the line with all of his body, putting all his weight onto his right hand, and he was asleep. (80–81)

In the same way as the Old Man had, I began to talk to my body and travel its infinite byways. This way, my fragility became a strength. A new way of being myself.

I could "forget" the cripple I had become.

I supplemented these routines — the meditation and mirror therapy — with theories being proposed in new research being done at the University of Victoria where they suggested that exercising your good or unaffected side was every bit as important for recovery as exercises prescribed for the damaged side. My half brother, Barrie, drew my attention to an article by Randy Shore that appeared in the *Vancouver Sun* on December 10, 2012:

Stroke victims recover use of weakened limbs by exercising unaffected limbs research finds

Stroke victims can make astonishing gains in strength in weakened limbs by training the unaffected limbs on the other side of their body, according to new research by the University of Victoria.

Neuroscientist Paul Zehr and PhD candidate Katie Dragert designed "ridiculously simple" devices made of wooden boards and cloth straps that stroke victims used to strengthen the muscles in their legs and ankles. Patients completed a six-week high-intensity training regime — not with the limbs weakened by the stroke, but with the limbs that were less affected or unaffected.

What happened surprised even the researchers.

Patients gained as much strength in the weakened leg as they did in the leg that did the exercises. Patients achieved strength gains of about 30 per cent in both the trained and untrained legs, a far more dramatic effect than previous research on healthy people had achieved.

The finding promises to be a boon to patients whose limb strength is so impaired by stroke that they can't lift or train the affected parts at all.

"Weakness is a big part of what happens after a stroke and if you can do something to increase people's strength, you can help them get walking . . . ," said Zehr.

Patients in the study suffered their stroke on average about 80 months before training. That suggests patients can benefit from the program years after a debilitating event.

Study participant Barb Oliver suffered from weakness in her left leg after a stroke 10 years ago, but continues to make gains through UVic's experimental programs.

"I couldn't walk at all and they didn't think I would ever walk again," said Oliver. "Now, I get around with a cane."

Zehr and Dragert employed a mostly forgotten 1894 discovery by Yale University researchers who found that when people train one arm, the other arm also gained strength.

"The arm that they trained got stronger, but the other arm got stronger, too, even though it wasn't trained," Zehr explained. "Over the years people have looked at cross-education of strength on different parts of the body, upper and lower limbs, and it pretty much shows up everywhere to a greater or lesser degree."

Most of the research found that the untrained limb gains about half as much strength as the trained limb.

"A 30-per-cent gain on the trained side usually results in a 15-per-cent gain on the untrained side," he said. "We thought that with all the damage caused by the stroke that we might see a five- or 10-per-cent gain in our patients' untrained limbs."

But the strength gains recorded in the UVic study of stroke victims were twice as high as the gains achieved by healthy people in past studies.

"Much of the training gain in strength and skill that people achieve through exercise takes place in the brain and the nervous system rather than the muscles themselves," Zehr said.

"The surprising strength of the cross-education effect suggests the training program may be tapping into communication pathways between the left and right sides of the brain and activating built-in — but little used — duplications in the neural wiring that controls movement," he said.

As soon as Pat read this article to me, I began doing exercises with my unaffected side. Everything about this rediscovered and revived research made perfectly good sense to me, because it targeted both the physical and mental effects of stroke. Simultaneously.

The principle was simple and commonsensical.

Simultaneity was the key.

Gradually, I was regaining minimal movement on my damaged side. For example, I was now able to transfer to my wheelchair with the aid of only one nurse instead of two. Deep down I knew if — by exercising my good side — I replicated the exercises that had already helped me regain some movement on my damaged side I should be able to accelerate my recovery. Even though it often felt like I was lifting or pushing air when I exercised my unaffected side, I persuaded myself that my unresponsive right side would react and relearn from my left side what was still possible: the dizzying heights of movement and the promise of a dreamed recovery.

According to recent research on brain plasticity discussed in Norman Doidge's *The Brain That Changes Itself*, the two halves of the brain are in more intimate contact than experts only a few years ago assumed to be the case. I'm convinced this connection is vital to successful stroke treatment. I'm confident the two hemispheres are in constant communication on pathways that criss-cross between the two halves of the brain. In fact, I'm convinced they're not separated at all; they are definitely integral parts of a whole.

So, I told myself, in ideal rehabilitation, the damaged side will register the movement of the good side and imitate or relearn what it's supposed to do. How simple and yet brilliant. A brain doing what comes to it naturally. What stroke survivors needed, as far as I could see, was guidance that married physiotherapy to neuroscience. Why had researchers abandoned what in 1894 seemed a simple and logical union?

Around noon, Owen arrived, like an affirmation.

Pat must have told me that he was coming, but in the busyness of therapy I had forgotten on which day.

Again.

All the different activities required so much concentration. And I seemed able to remember only a limited number of appointment times before they blurred into one another. I was constantly turning up in the wrong room. Late. This was a common mistake made by all the patients, but for the most part no one took any notice. Occasionally you would see a therapist prowling the halls in search of a patient.

But sometimes, forgetting can be a virtue and an advantage. When Owen walked through the door behind his mother, I didn't have to feign surprise. I was, as the Brits would say, gobsmacked. And delighted. Immediately I felt a surge of love, much as I had on the day Nicole had arrived. From both of them I felt as though I were the recipient of some sort of special healing hormone. Sitting there in my wheelchair, I couldn't help smiling, even though I immediately worried that he would see me as a wounded animal. As a creature that was less than human. Again, I have no idea why I felt this way. Perhaps it was pride, but I think it had more to do with the way we cling to our own youth, to an image of ourselves that has more to do with memory than mirrors.

He sauntered into the room then cut around Pat and gave me a hug.

"You look good," he said, "much better than I expected."

I wasn't quite sure how to take that. What had he expected? All sorts of monstrous images popped into my mind. Did he think I would be comatose or a hollow, grey body with spittle dripping off my chin or a pathetic figure whose sense of self had receded so far into the past it would take an autopsy to discover the cause? I had to admit that for a few days that's exactly how I had felt.

Sensing my unease, he said: "You're up and Mom says you're starting to do some therapy. Actually getting some movement back. From what I've heard, that's light years ahead of a week ago."

"Yes," I said, "I suppose it is, but recovery is very slow. Imperceptible, at least from where I lie in bed most of the time." I was beginning to feel the tears well up in my eyes, not because of anything I was telling him, but because he was there, in the room. With me and his mother. "And the pain, at times, is excruciating, especially when I suffer spasms. My leg and foot twist inward as if clamped in some medieval contraption used to torture heretics. And if I'm lucky, my arm and hand will shudder at the same time and vibrate like a tuning fork. You have no idea."

He started to respond, but I interrupted him: "And I speak funny. Can you understand me?"

My mouth curved down like a comma interrupting my next thought.

Why was I whining? He had travelled so far to be with me, from Dease Lake, a seven-hour drive down the Cassiar Highway, which started five hundred miles north of Vancouver and ran parallel to the Alaska Panhandle to Terrace. Through bear, wolf, elk and moose country, in the middle of nowhere. Landmarks were rivers and mountains, not buildings, obelisks, towers, museums, galleries, piazzas. And then by plane to Vancouver.

"I'm sorry," I said, "I shouldn't be complaining. How's Jen? How was your trip? It's so good to see you. So good," I repeated.

I wanted to ask him to give me another hug, but I was afraid that I might be asking for too much. I mustn't get carried away, I thought.

"I can understand you well enough," he said. "There's just a hint of a slur. Not bad, though."

He folded his arms across his chest, and then his right hand moved up to his chin and he caressed his new beard. Thoughtfully. Carefully considering what to say next. Fidgeting. Owen had never known what to do with his hands.

"It's really good to see you as well," he said. "I only wish I'd been able to get here sooner."

Now when I looked at him he was much bigger than I remembered. Taller and definitely more muscular. He was a big man. Handsome. When had this transformation taken place? Along with two friends from the UK, Edwin and Mary Webb, Pat and I had only just visited him and his partner, Jen, this past summer on our way to the Yukon and over the "Top of the World Highway" to Alaska. Why hadn't I noticed at that time who he had become? Was I that blind? Or was deliberate evasion a form of reprieve many of us construct in order to ignore the passage of time and the inevitability of our own deaths? A "hold" button of sorts.

For five straight days he came to me, arriving shortly after breakfast and remaining until around four in the afternoon. On two of those days his mother stayed home. We both agreed that she had some healing of her own to do. And some well-earned downtime to take. At this stage, not even her beauty could outlast the grind of constant concern and naked fear. The stress on caregivers, we agreed, must be shattering. Pat looked fagged — almost like an old woman — her skin beginning to wrinkle as if all the threads that held her together had suddenly come unravelled. No matter how strong the person, no matter how secure they feel in their relationship, everything in a caregiver's world is turned upside down and inside out the instant a partner or friend suffers a stroke. In a matter of seconds, routines, beliefs, dreams, hopes and memories can vaporize and confidence vanish.

Each day, from the minute he walked through the door, Owen would ask me how my night had gone. Had I slept well? Had I experienced any pain? Had I had any dark thoughts? Had I eaten enough breakfast? Rapidly. Yes (relatively), yes, no (not that I had dwelt on), yes, I answered. He seemed especially concerned about my emotional well-being. I was sure Pat had spoken to him about those moments when I became morose, when I felt naked and raw and tearful. I appreciated his concern, but I had taken a vow: to remain positive and happy. And recover.

Once he was convinced I was all right he would finish getting me ready for therapy. At first he had wanted to give me a shave, but I told him I had decided to grow a beard. A seasonal thing, I told him. Besides, a beard was more convenient, was much easier for me to manage on my own.

Okay, he nodded.

I could tell he was keen to get started, more so than I was. Chatting away, he pushed me down the hall to the gym and did what he could to assist the physiotherapist. When she had me tottering along on a walker, he followed with the wheelchair, always on the ready to catch me if and when I toppled backwards. We became a merry little troupe flitting from one piece of gym equipment to another.

"Your muscles have atrophied badly," Deena said to me. "We need to do some simple exercises to strengthen them. Don't be alarmed, but it's going to be difficult at first. And take time. You won't be able to do any of the things that used to come to you instinctively."

Everyone kept stressing time, kept reminding me of the length of *time* recovery was going to take. This obsession seemed ironic to me. Weren't the able-bodied people the ones chasing the clock? Weren't they the ones obsessed with schedules and appointments? From where I sat in my wheelchair, time moved at a crawl, and during the night hours, when I dreamt about movement, time came to a standstill.

Longingly, I took a glance through the row of windows that ran the length of the gym. Even on this grey day I felt impatient, a need to escape my incarceration before it smothered me. Outside, large, wet snowflakes landed on the pavement and melted. Soon the snow would stick. For the moment, I decided, I was better off where I was, learning to walk again.

All in good time! I thought. All in good time.

"Let's get started," Owen said.

From the beginning, Owen's message was positive. So positive it put a shine on a rather gloomy day. Nicole had recently told me a story she'd heard from a friend who had attended a conference with First Nations women about policing in the north. Many of the stories about police treatment of First Nations people were horrific, but one elder spoke of a young policeman in her area who approached conflicts or domestic disputes with kindness, understanding and words. Always words. Sometimes humour. He would separate the feuding parties and say, "We'll talk about it in the morning. Okay?" There was no blame. No one demeaned. He treated everyone with equal respect. Hearing this story, Nicole's friend was curious, knowing already that Nicole's brother was stationed in the region. When Nicole's friend asked the elder if she knew the name of the policeman, she had replied, "Yes, Owen."

Nicole had smiled and said, "My brother, possibly."

I was not surprised. Slightly pensive, yes, but pleased. Hugely pleased. What else would a policeman with a degree in Classics do but talk? He had a wealth of lessons from Greek and Roman poetry, philosophy and drama on which to draw.

Over the years, Owen's and my relationship had changed. In my mind he had finally grown up. During his adolescent years we'd had our share of disagreements and misunderstandings. Not a particularly unique situation. Now, from what I could see, there were fewer all-night parties and fewer careless spending sprees. Naturally he would disagree with my characterization. He would say things hadn't changed all that much. And likely he was right. He still enjoyed travelling when the whim hit, and he figured if he could indulge a fantasy he would. Flying to Chicago on a weekend to attend both a basketball game and a baseball game was, in his mind, not only possible but would be a terrible missed opportunity — not to mention financially irresponsible — if not taken. A short holiday on the Croatian coast in the middle of winter was a matter of personal health and sanity. In a way he was the free spirit I had once intended to be. Perhaps I was jealous or perhaps I had become more tolerant and forgiving. Or maybe I had finally learned patience. I didn't know.

What seemed more probable was that each of us had learned to love the other for what the other was. At times, though, he still looked at me as if I were sporting two heads.

One day after I had been served lunch in my room, I sprawled out on the bed. The fatigue I felt from what seemed like minimal exercise had numbed my brain. My right side was hopelessly knotted up and in pain. I was exhausted. I listened to Owen, his voice soothing, wrapping around me like a fine mist. Whatever he had to say had to be inserted between my frequent naps and Jack yelling out one of his "Bird" calls.

Owen talked about his job (sometimes mind-bogglingly scary, I thought), about the LA Clippers (a team he'd followed since he was a teenager playing high school basketball), about living in the north, about Jen and their plans to get married next year, and about his desire to get a posting back on the coast so they could be closer to us. He missed the rainforest. Hearing this news sent me soaring.

I liked the idea that he would be able to help his mother with the heavy work in the garden. Digging, and climbing a stepladder into fruit trees to do the pruning.

So far, since his arrival, Pat said he'd cooked all the evening meals. He's a pretty good chef, she added, on the spicy side. And on his second night he'd taken her to see the latest James Bond flick. *Skyfall* with Daniel Craig. Her choice.

I know we discussed other, more serious subjects, but I forget the details now. What mattered was that these man-to-man, heart-to-heart talks relaxed me, made me realize how fortunate I was to have a son and daughter, my own flesh and blood, who loved us enough to want to take care of us. I was pleased to know they both had a driving need to give.

Two other major events took place while Owen was visiting.

First, my half-brothers, Barrie with his wife Karen, Brian with his wife Barb, and Guy, had brought my eighty-seven-year-old mother for a long-anticipated visit. With Owen and Pat this made nine of us sitting around the tables in the multi-purpose room. Soon Barrie was talking about one of his many interests, likely about food or books. I don't recall. Like many people he probably wanted to talk to fill up a situation that he found awkward and personally worrying. Brian slipped uncomfortably behind a wall of silence. Guy told jokes. I think most of us find a way to hide our worry. But all I remember is drifting off, partly because I was plum tired and partly because words tended to become jumbled in my brain and rearrange themselves in a verbal stew. Sleeping was a matter of self-defence. I do recall being extremely happy to see them all but also finding the experience overwhelming. There was simply too much to take in.

My hearing at the time was amplified and would continue to be so for months, and when too many voices spoke at once I became anxious. Later, when I was out of therapy, I would begin to gasp for air and search for escape routes as soon as I felt confined or trapped in a crowd. Restaurants were the worst, when the chatter at nearby tables would mingle and reach a crescendo that I thought would smother me. Sound tightened around my head like a wooden vice and threatened to squeeze the life out of me.

As I looked from face to face, everyone seemed serious. Grave. Fearful. Although I sensed tenderness and compassion from all of them, they were also predictably cautious, not wanting to transgress some undefined boundary, like a no man's land, that separated the living from the "undead," of which I was one. I knew they wished me well, of that I had no doubt, but for some reason their caution made me feel like a curiosity. Isolated and alone. I desperately wanted to be with them, and yet I felt like the dead parrot in a *Monty Python* skit. The butt of some grotesque gag.

I began to slouch in my wheelchair, my body sagged. Like an accordion when the air was released. I remember being embarrassed by my wheelchair, by my dependence on it. I wanted to be like them, sitting on a wooden chair, not the "cripple" I was, restrained in this vinyl and metal appendage. I realized at that moment that sometimes you can't help the way you see yourself. You form an image of who or what you are and for better or worse that's what you become. I didn't like the persona I'd conjured, but I seemed to be stuck with it.

Minutes later, my mother, who was sitting next to me, leaned in and whispered, "How are you doing?"

"I'm fine," I said, but her eyes read me differently.

"Okay," I added.

She frowned. "Be honest," she said.

"As well as can be expected," I continued, trying desperately to paint a portrait of someone who was bold and self-assured.

"I don't believe you," she said in a friendly way. "You look tired to me."

I glanced around the circle of familiar faces. She was right. I wasn't handling this very well. Perhaps there were too many of them, as tactless and as ungrateful as this must sound.

"Yes," I said to her, my voice barely audible, "I am tired. Very tired."

While friends and family who came to see me over these weeks were an inspiration to recovery, providing much-needed relief from the monotony of the hospital routine, I learned from the family visit that numbers mattered. I could take only so much attention

and interrogation. From early morning, before sunrise, until bedtime, the parade of people in and out of the room was endless —
nurses, doctors, therapists, kitchen staff, cleaners, visitors. Putting
on a suitable face, whether it was a welcoming smile or the composed face of the dutiful patient, required energy and chutzpah. I
lacked both.

I realized there was a limit to the number of people I could see at
any given time throughout the day.

Oddly enough, apart from Pat, the only other person who was a
daily visitor to my room during my five weeks as an in-patient in
therapy was Des, the cleaner. Every morning, just after breakfast, he
came into the room with his mop, brooms, sprays, rags, buckets and
sponges and began his cleaning ritual. Even in the early days on rehab, when I still sounded like I was speaking through a mouthful of
marbles, we jabbered on about hockey, football, his kids, my family,
his upcoming trip to Hawaii, a new recipe he'd tried out on his
family, his wife, how fast he was on skates and so on. He could have
been a pro, he said, if he hadn't been so small and short.

Any subject could get him started. Des loved talking and he could
lean on any mop or broom handle for good stretches of time. Every
so often he would make a motion, a little swirl, which gave the impression that he was hard at work. I'm convinced we had spots that
were the cleanest in the hospital.

The other thing about Des was that he always smiled and laughed.
And he called each of us by our first name. This familiarity was
significant. He treated every patient as if they were a friend, as if
they had some role and importance in his life. We weren't just in-
mates in an asylum for the terminally handicapped. We mattered.
Periodically he would turn to Jack and say "Bird" and the two men
would smile conspiratorially. Comrades in some sort of confederacy.
To Des we were as human as anyone else.

Thankfully most of the nurses shared Des's sense of empathy. A
couple of the younger nurses were a bit brusque and tossed off a

patient's distress signal with a shake of the head and a "heigh-ho, can't you see I'm busy." The truth was some nurses, like some visitors, were more congenial, more cheerful than others. Most made a positive contribution to recovery while a few descended on the tiny part of the world that patients occupied like the unholy duo of "doom and gloom." But the majority of the nurses were angels, as far as I was concerned, Cheryl and Ann Marie in particular, who were not only passionate about nursing but allowed brief glimpses into their own lives as a part of the healing process. Cheryl told me about the acreage she and her husband had bought on a lake in the interior, somewhere in the Chilcotin, in bear and moose country, where they "chilled out" in front of a fire on weekends. A simpler life. Ann Marie wrote poetry and over Christmas was off to Casablanca on a writing retreat.

The other event that Owen played a role in had nothing to do with my stroke. A month before my brain was blitzed I had undergone my second cataract surgery and the follow-up appointment had been scheduled for the morning of November 30. This was a routine examination to make sure the surgery had been successful. To me this first excursion outside the confines of the hospital seemed totally unnecessary. I felt as if my eyes and ears were the only working parts of my body. I didn't want to go anywhere, certainly not out into the slushy snow.

As Owen pushed me through the automatic sliding doors, I realized how tropical our ward felt. Even though I was now wrapped in my heavy winter coat, an icy gust of wind cut through my clothing, right to the bone. I shivered, my skin covered in goose bumps, and I asked if we could turn back. Pat said no: getting out would be good for me.

The ophthalmologist's office was across the street from the hospital through an intersection. When the light turned green and the little stick man flashed for us to proceed, I could feel the pity from drivers sitting behind the steering wheels of their cars, watching me. Not one pedestrian walking towards me would look me in the eye. They preferred for me to be invisible. Blink, and as if by magic, I'd disappear.

In the ophthalmologist's office the treatment I received was much the same. Everyone avoided eye contact; some looked at the wheelchair as if it were a relic from a horror movie. I was one of the zombie survivors, wheeling about searching for other victims. My kin, my ilk. The receptionist, who couldn't see me over the counter, spoke to Pat who gave her all my details. Apparently I was unable to answer for myself.

With a little assistance I managed the transfer from my wheelchair to the doctor's fancy examination chair. Without noting a change in my status, he examined my eye and pronounced me good to go.

"I've had a stroke since the surgery," I said.

He paused, ready to move on to his next patient.

"I noticed," he said. "You look like you're doing well. Keep up the good work. Your eyes are first-rate. 20/20."

For some reason I felt cheated.

I didn't know what to say. Wasn't this what I wanted? To be treated as normal?

Yet I couldn't wait to get back to my room in rehab.

Seek a safe place away from the depths people sometimes sink to when they feel lost or forgotten, Owen had said. When he talked about his job, he said: It's too easy to be pulled down by someone else's misery. Let yourself be drawn into the light, into the infinite lifetimes each of us faces as a possibility. Right now, rest and recovery should be at the forefront of your thoughts, he reminded me.

"You can never take what you witness personally, whether at an accident scene, a domestic dispute, a crime of passion or a murder. Otherwise you'll be overwhelmed and become jaded. Any 'sense' life might make then, becomes obscured," he told me, stopping to reflect. His back stiffening. "Compassion is one thing," he continued, looking me directly in the eyes, "but you have to make a choice between the passive resignation of some of the other patients and your own determination to recover."

But what about Jack? I wondered after Owen had gone back home to Dease Lake where the temperature frequently dropped below minus fifty degrees — Celsius or Fahrenheit didn't seem to matter when I considered how cold that was.

I already missed his conversation and guidance.

What about Jack, then? Jack the "Bird Man." I had been studying Jack for three weeks, since my arrival on the rehab floor. From opposite sides of the room we watched each other, him me as if he were witnessing through me how he had come to be where he was; me him because I wasn't convinced he was the "poor mindless soul," totally lost to dementia, that everyone thought him to be. I heard whispers that shortly he was to be moved to a place where "hopeless" cases were sent. But there were times when I thought I glimpsed a man who at times was every bit as lucid as the rest of us. And there were times when he smiled and winked at me as if he knew a secret about the desires men have that he wanted to share with me. Behind his gaze, though, there was always an element of suspicion. Understandably so, given the way he was often treated.

Yes, I rang for the nurse when he couldn't find his buzzer and he yelled out "Bird" repeatedly, but that was because the cord had somehow managed to get caught up in his bedding or wrapped around his arm or he was in excruciating pain. And then he was helpless.

"Bird" got a response!

Jack confirmed my belief that a lot of patients floundered in despair and finally gave up because the diagnosis they were given didn't present recovery as a choice. As I say, most therapy was physical, not cognitive, so unless patients could get out of bed and find a way to cope with their depression and mental fatigue, they were not likely to receive constructive help. If they were coasting down-hill and could see little in their future, they would likely enter free fall. They would be left to cope with the place where they landed. And without a supportive family, they would be alone.

When I had free time away from therapy, I sprawled out on my bed and slept. By this time, with a little effort, I could make the transfer from my wheelchair to the bed without assistance. Outside the window, just beyond the parking lot, there was an old Japanese cherry tree — a marvellous twisted sculpture reaching wildly into the winter sky — leafless at this time of the year. Skeletal, the tree looked like a charcoal drawing of an apparition. Presaging what? Early in the New Year it would don glorious pink blossoms, pro-claiming its ardour for the renewal of life.

For a few weeks I had also been watching Jack perform for the speech therapist. She sat beside him or at the foot of the bed, de-pending on Jack's angle of sight, and displayed cards for him. His task was to identify what was on the card.

"Come on, Jack, what do you see?"

He lifted his arm, pushed his thick glasses up his nose with his index finger, and tried to focus on the card through one level of his trifocals.

"Car."

"Good, and this one?"

"House."

"And this one?"

"Tree."

"Excellent. Very good. You're doing better than you did yester-day."

In response to this last comment, I watched Jack tense up, briefly, obviously annoyed, and then his face became expressionless. When the therapist revealed the next card he rolled his head and said "Bird," slightly louder than he had answered before.

"Jack, don't be stubborn. You know what it is." She was already upset with him. I don't remember now how many times I watched this little drama unfold. But he then looked at her severely as if at an idiot who was missing an important part of the puzzle.

"Bird, bird, bird," he answered as if a warbler snapping at an annoying fly. If he noticed me watching he would give me a quick grin.

Exhausted and defensive — sometimes her mood was difficult to figure out — the therapist would rise, collect her things and mince out of the room. When she returned to her office she would likely write DEMENTED into his file.

Undaunted, Jack settled back to enjoy his newly won peace, his release from what he perceived as mindless repetition. Here was an example of the infantilization of a man who, though silenced and manacled, still had an inner life as a mature person with wit and perspective. Although, admittedly, no one knew for sure. At first I imagined the tests aroused his wistful curiosity but as time passed I thought they probably became intrusive and annoying, perhaps a reminder of unwanted authority.

When his wife visited, which was infrequent, she never stayed longer than half an hour. Apparently she had a great distance to travel. Ladysmith was thirty kilometres south of the city, and she didn't drive. Public transit was out of the question. Often she came with a friend, who presumably drove, and she would immediately tell Jack that the two of them had planned an afternoon of shopping. She would have to leave soon. He would grunt, nod his head and give her a pained but forgiving look.

I noticed his wife yelled at him and he cringed as if he were being chastised. No matter what the disability, some people feel they have to shout at all disabled people. She was one of those. Eventually Jack injected "Bird" into their conversation and she turned to her friend and raised her eyebrows as if she had been snubbed or offended in some way.

"Why do you have to say that?" she asked quietly, and Jack eyed her as if he'd caught a glimpse of a ghost. Perhaps the rascally boy he'd once been.

"Bird," he repeated. "Bird."

And suddenly, after a curt "by your leave" and a peck on the cheek, she left.

One day after lunch I sat daydreaming in my wheelchair. Lately the atmosphere in the room had become much more hopeful. And cheerful. Both of the amputees had been fitted with prosthetics and both were beginning to see the prospect of walking again. And returning home — without being too much of a burden.

I turned from looking out the window to see Jack watching me. His gaze, in spite of the hell his life had become, was playful and inquisitive. Up until now, all of our communication had been across the width of the room. Usually monosyllabic. Or with gestures. Now he seemed to be beckoning me. So I rolled across the room to the side of his bed. He looked down on me and smiled.

"Jack," he said. "My name's Jack, although some call me John."

"Yes," I said, "I know. They have John on the nameplate outside the door."

"Oh, they would. More formal."

I nodded.

"I want to tell you a story. I'm eighty-four. Not that that matters to anyone." He hesitated as if considering a small regret. "Everyone's in a rush these days." Pause. "Do you have some free time?"

"My next therapy session's at 1:30," I told him.

"Good," he said. "This won't take long. Besides, like you, I get tired quickly."

He gave me a quick glance to see if I was still paying attention.

"I was born on a farm." He sighed and spread his hands, as if releasing a carrier pigeon into the sky. "It was the happiest time of my life . . ."

And then he went on to tell me about his life as a kid on a farm. About trudging through the mud in gumboots to herd the cows back to the barn, and then milking them. About fetching eggs from the henhouse. And helping his dad till the fields behind a plough horse. He loved that horse, a gentle giant of an animal. About meals made with vegetables grown in the family's own garden. About apples, plums and pears picked, preserved and stored for the winter in the root cellar, along with potatoes, carrots, turnips, beets and onions. A taste of summer when the snows came. About stacking wood for the stove, harvested from the treed area at the bottom of the property, near the creek. Alder, mostly. He told me about swinging on a rope tied to a beam in the barn and landing softly on the recently harvested hay. On and on he went, excited to have an audience, although I could see he was tiring.

As though spreading seed by hand, he often tossed "Bird" into his story. I found this habit as puzzling and as annoying as everyone else did. Why did he do this? Was he being intentionally obstinate? Then, when I thought about the context, an idea flashed into my brain. Why hadn't I considered this before? I asked him if he meant "tractor" or "bale" or "pressure cooker" after he had said "Bird" and he smiled and answered, "Yes, yes, that's it. That's the word."

The mistake the speech therapist was making was that she had been taught a procedure that included certain specific steps, and when Jack didn't respond accordingly she assumed that he was slowly losing his mind. That he was a lost soul. She was well-intentioned, but her training hadn't taught her to find the "human being" that was Jack. Every stroke is unique and haphazard, I repeated to myself. There was a simple answer to Jack's use of "Bird." When he got to a place in his tale where he couldn't remember the correct word, partly because he was too tired, he used "Bird" in its place. "Bird" could mean or be anything. He knew exactly what he wanted to say; sometimes he simply couldn't find the right word for the particular occasion.

"I should never have left the farm. I wasn't cut out to be a 'Bird,'" he said. For some reason I think he became an insurance salesman.

As I rolled down the hall to mirror therapy and passed room after room of bedridden patients, I wondered how many of them were like Jack, abandoned, not out of any gross incompetence or negligence but because so little was known about the brain. How many were like Jean-Dominique Bauby and "locked in," unable to speak their mind? They were living inside their strokes. Each one unique! Each one trying to find the person everyone else assumed was lost.

Memory.

Memory sustained me, especially through the long nights as an in-patient in a room where voices inspired flights of the imagination.

Memory became a lifeline. But to what?

A past, apprehensive about a future?

How was remembering helping me?

Which reality did it represent?

As I have noted and repeat, Joshua Foer in *Moonwalking with Einstein* says: "For all the advances that have been made in recent decades, it's still the case that no one has ever actually seen a memory in the human brain." (34) A little later on in this wonderful exploration of remembering, he also suggests our earliest reliable memories take us back, at best, to age three or four:

> Until the age of three or four, almost nothing that happens to us leaves the sort of lasting impression that can be consciously recalled as an adult. The average age that people report having their earliest memory is three and a half, and those tend to be just blurry, fragmentary snapshots that are often false. How strange that during the period when a person is learning more rapidly than at any other point in his life — when one is learning to walk and talk and make sense of the world — so little of that learning is of the kind that is explicitly memorable. (84)

And yet, two to three weeks into my stay in rehab, I was transported back to a time near the beginning of my own life, when *I* was first making sense of the world.

While lying in my hospital bed one evening, wedged between mountains of pillows, I experienced one of the most profound moments of my life. At two in the morning, I awoke from a dream in which I remembered a memory that predated anything I had previously known. Prior to this, the earliest recollection I could summon was from around age five or six, but this post-stroke memory took me back years, to around eleven months. The image was vivid, as detail after detail gathered in my consciousness like an archaeologist's reconstruction of an ancient ruin.

I had been taken by my adoptive mother to a photographer's studio in New Westminster. To a storefront on the main street, near the Fraser River, I think. Columbia Street, where cars, mostly black, were parked diagonally. Near my grandfather's veterinarian practice, which I would visit later. In fact, he may have been the one to deliver us to the studio. The studio was dimly lit and damp except for the bright lights near the back wall set up around a stage or table surrounded by dark curtains. Startled by the glare, I began to cry. Uncontrollably. I bawled my eyes out.

I was dressed in a cream-coloured knitted outfit — sweater, shorts and socks — my mother had bought or possibly knit, especially for the occasion. The photograph itself, which I have framed and standing on a dresser, tells me this much of the story.

Why was I being so difficult? I imagine I was scared. She, I recalled, had no idea how to comfort me. I remembered being held under the armpits at arm's length and being scrutinized as if I were counterfeit. The photographer seemed to be in a hurry and extremely impatient. Perhaps annoyed. Was it because of my lack of cooperation? I remembered his suspenders. His rolled-up sleeves. His vest and tie. The long room with a dark, wooden-plank floor, wainscotting and no windows on either side.

Then there was a moment when I was distracted — was it by a

toy waved at me or the photographer snapping his fingers? — and the tears stopped. A flash of light bounced off screens, white umbrellas, and blinded me. I sensed my mother's relief, and heard her nervous laughter. The embarrassment. The apologies.

As I lay there in the hospital I was amazed by the clarity of these images from so long ago. Where had they come from and why now? How much of what I recalled was imagined or revised? And how far into the past could I see?

Did my stroke jolt something loose?

Was this merely a fragment of memory, chipped free of context, drifting about aimlessly in my brain? In my fatigue was I making associations that never existed? Was I writing fiction based on hearsay and invention? In short, gossip-become-story. What else was there? Was this the way we remembered our ancestors?

And yet the images were so real.

I remembered other events with equal clarity, from a little later, but from before age three. I felt like I was on a salvage mission. I remembered going over the handlebars of my tricycle and smashing forehead first into the cement sidewalk. I remembered seeing stars and experiencing dizziness not unlike the confusion I had experienced with the stroke.

Over the next weeks and months, I heard or read other accounts from stroke survivors who experienced improved memory in the wake of their stroke. What role might these changes to memory or this improved memory have on stroke recovery?

I needed to know if accessing such memories would in some way assist me with remapping my brain. I was tired of feeling helpless. I wanted to know if I was finding a new me. The "deeper me" that the yogic tradition seeks to experience. Pure being, pure consciousness, pure bliss. *Sat-cit-ānanda*. With normal pathways knocked out, I was free to discover novel ways of being in the world. These choices seemed limitless. A random stream-of-consciousness journey had considerable appeal. Or was I on a futile quest?

A year after my release from out-patient therapy, I read an article in the University of Leeds alumni magazine about Dr. Richard Allen, a member of the Faculty of Medicine and Health at the university who was doing interesting research into memory. I wrote to him, hoping he might be able to help me to understand how memory might be altered after any form of brain trauma.

April 1, 2014

Dear Richard Allen,

I read about your research in the Leeds alumni on-line magazine with interest. I'm a 1970 graduate of Leeds in English. In November of 2012, at the age of 69, I suffered a serious ischemic stroke to my right side. While the entire damaged side of my body was paralyzed, my cognitive abilities were not affected. In fact, if anything they were enhanced, especially my memory. And in particular my long-term memory. While I was in hospital, I recalled events from my life from as early as 11 months. Prior to the stroke my earliest memory was from around age 5. I have been able to verify these very early memories through relatives and archives. In addition to improved memory, my senses, hearing and sight in particular, became much more acute.

Of course, I have a theory why this enhancement happened. I was wondering if your research has looked into the effects of brain trauma on memory? I've been reading some of the most recent literature on the subject but I'd be interested in any thoughts you might have. Three of the most useful books I've read are *Moonwalking with Einstein*, *The Brain that Changes Itself* and *The Future of the Mind*.

Thanks for your attention.

Best wishes,
Ron Smith

April 3, 2014

Dear Ron,

Thank you for your email. I was very interested to read
about your experiences.

I personally have not researched the impact of brain trauma
on memory, though I'm not familiar with any previous cases
from the literature of improved early memory retrieval
following stroke. This serves to make your experiences more
interesting, of course. As you say, prior to the stroke, your
earliest memories were from around age 5; this is very
common, and indeed even Freud talked about childhood
'amnesia' (though we've rather moved on from Freud's
explanations of this, of course). It would be very interesting
to know what kinds of memories you recollected from early
life, in terms of the type of event and detail associated with
them.

I take it that, based on your web address below, you are
based in Canada? Whereabouts would you be?

Best wishes
Richard

April 3, 2014

Dear Richard,

Thanks for your prompt reply. Yes, I'm based in Canada,
on Vancouver Island, north of Nanaimo in a place called
Nanoose Bay.

I gather from the reading I've done that some people are able to recall events from an age as early as 3 1/2, but this is rare. As you say, Freud aside, I gather contemporary theory still holds to the idea that for most of us memory begins around ages 5/6. Certainly that was the case for me. As I'm sure you know, one of the side effects of a stroke is a loss of self, physically and cognitively. Over time there were several things I could not remember how to do or objects I recognized but did not know how to use. For example, when a therapist placed some play dough on a table in front of me, along with a knife and fork, and asked me to pretend I was eating, I immediately picked up the fork but not the knife. I recognized both objects, but for the life of me I couldn't remember how to use the knife.

In the initial stages of my stroke I was fed intravenously, consequently after a few days I felt extremely hungry. This had two outcomes. I had decided that to hold on to my identity I needed to recall who I was through memories. This was a very deliberate act. I have no idea why I chose to do this. I just seemed to sense that it would help. By association, one of the first memories I visited was a time in my life when I went for a lengthy stretch without food. A period in the 1960s, when I was bumming around Europe and ran out of money. I would slip in and out of this memory as a way of coping with my present hunger and as a reminder of who I was.

Then one night, two to three weeks into my stroke, I woke up with a vivid recollection of having my baby picture taken. I could see the room; I remembered the photographer, the lights, my crying, the photographer's frustration, etc, everything in amazing detail. I thought the photograph had been taken when I was about 1 1/2. I later talked to an older cousin who corrected me and said the photo was taken at 11 months. My age was not a part of the memory. The photographer, she told me, was her grandfather on the maternal side, a man I saw only that one time. She was quite surprised by what I could recall of his studio and him. I had a few other memories of this sort but as I started to recover they became less frequent. Oh, I should mention that I was adopted at about this time so I suspect my brain had already registered this event as fairly traumatic.

From what I've read, recent theory proposes that forgetting is part of the brain's function. Perhaps a defence against overload. With a stroke those defences can be knocked out. I think this may have something to do with experiencing those early memories. I'd be interested in hearing what you think might have happened.

Best wishes,
Ron

■

April 22, 2014

Dear Ron,

I found your email really interesting, so thank you for sharing some of your experiences. A number of thoughts struck me as I was reading your email, and while I'm by no means an expert in long-term memory and forgetting (my research focus is more on the short-term, or working memory), you might find them useful to consider.

– Memory is represented across the brain, so as you found, after impacts such as those caused by stroke, it can divide in strange (but often predictable) ways, with some knowledge and experience intact and other information slower to return.

– The self is an important concept, and may be intimately connected to memory. Indeed, the dominant theory in the field of autobiographical memory is that our sense of self is based on our memories, and vice versa. I have a PhD student who is currently examining this relationship in healthy young adults and clinical groups, including people with dementia and acquired brain injury. We don't know as much about this relationship in people who have experienced a stroke, but your views are very useful and informative. I'd be happy to tell you more about this work (or indeed, have my student do so, as she is the expert!).

– Traumatic memories tend to be particularly well represented and accessible (more so than neutral memories), for a variety of possible reasons (possibly related to self concept, but also perhaps the close relationship between the brain areas responsible for forming new long-term memories and those for processing emotion).

– It is likely the case that some memories are not success-fully consolidated, and so are never properly stored in long-term memory. Others may be gradually lost over time. We don't know for sure whether memories are truly forgotten, or simply become inaccessible, so it is possible that you have been able to gain new access to memories, or fragments of memory, that were previously inaccessible.

– It is also worth bearing in mind the recent view of episodic memory as being constructive and reconstructive in nature. This view states that when we remember, we do not reactivate a precise record of what previously happened; instead, we rebuild the memory anew every time, using sensory information and knowledge about ourselves, the world, and the context of the original event. It might be worth thinking about some of your experiences from this perspective?

If you are interested in reading around the subject, I'd recommend Charles Fernyhough's *Pieces of Light*, which is a very readable introduction to the modern science of memory. Charles is a novelist as well as a neuropsychologist, so this text is very accessible.

By the sound of it, you are likely familiar with some of
these ideas already, but hopefully this is of some interest.

Best wishes,
Richard

Although I have no evidence to support my theory, I believe now
and have since the night of that early memory, that my stroke essentially knocked out my various defence systems. The regulator/
governor was gone, all the filters wiped out. Certainly immediately
after the stroke my senses were heightened, especially my sight
and hearing, I became very emotionally vulnerable, and I suddenly
seemed able to access memories that were dormant, hidden, or, I
had assumed, lost forever. I'm convinced our brains develop various
ways of protecting us from experiencing cognitive overload, which
I suspect would drive us crazy if we went about unprotected in our
day-to-day lives. Michio Kaku in *The Future of the Mind* talks about
forgetting as one of the main survival tools we have to cope with
potential meltdown. The ability to make rapid selections and choices,
I believe, is another.

After my stroke I felt bombarded. For several weeks I felt as if I
was under attack, through my senses as well as my thoughts. I remember growing very weary, a typical response to stroke, but also
wishing people would stop talking. Thoughts on any subject,
whether spoken or written, presented too many alternatives (another reason for my not reading). So much seemed to be happening.
What I had done automatically in the past now occupied my brain
with every little detail. It was no longer just a matter of getting up,
getting dressed and going out; I now had to think my way through
each step.

In other words, I believe what we develop as routine is one of our
refined defence systems. With the stroke, routine vanished. Increasingly I found it very difficult to make decisions. If offered choices, I
didn't know what to do. I went on "selection overload." I would
mull over solutions until every one seemed plausible. Faced with a

decision — and this went on for months — I would glance around, search for an answer, hoping to find it etched on some tablet or written in the ether, find nothing, hang my head and withdraw into some remote corner of my imagined universe. Not only was I unable to make a decision, I didn't *want* to make one. Making a choice meant a flood of possibilities, far too many with which to cope.

Memory plays a huge role in all of our actions. What to remember and what to forget makes it possible for us to get through the day. In those first weeks after my stroke it was almost as if I remembered too much. In a way, memory immobilized me. And yet, as I said earlier, memory was the one reliable way I found to hold on to who I was, to regain identity. In retrospect, this irony was the perfect Catch-22.

I wrote back to Richard outlining these thoughts and he kindly responded to me with the following:

September 18, 2014

Dear Ron,

Apologies, I was speaking at a major conference during July (the International Conference on Working Memory, held in Cambridge) and these things tend to dominate attention for a while! I was then away in France on an enjoyable though rainy holiday. I hope you had a good summer.

You raise several interesting points in your email of July 9th. One thing that strikes me is your discussion of a regulator, governor, or filter being wiped out, and this leading to difficulty coping with too much memory and sensory information. The ability to control, regulate, and inhibit information is thought to be a key aspect of what is termed 'executive function'. This inhibitory control ability is broadly based within the frontal lobes, and is important for helping us control automatic responses to situations, focus on information in the environment, and keep on top of information retrieved from long-term memory. It has been shown to develop through childhood and may decline with healthy ageing, and is often disrupted as a result of brain injury. I wouldn't want to offer this as a firm explanation obviously, but it's worth considering.

One well-known case that you might find relevant is that of Jill Price, a lady who was described as having 'hyperthymestic syndrome'. She reports that she is constantly bombarded with autobiographical memories. I've attached the original article describing her case here (she was initially described as patient AJ). The causes of her problems remain controversial, but it is worth noting that she seems to have some executive problems that might be related to trouble inhibiting her recollections. I'm far from an expert on her case though!

Your noting of problems making choices is also interesting. This could be related again to this issue of executive function (decision-making very much draws on EF). It also, as you say, relates to memory, as we often make decisions and plan future actions based on our memories of past events.

On the broader issue of whether these points relate to your memory for very early lifetime events, I wouldn't like to speculate too much. As I said previously, research generally tends to suggest that we are not able to recollect these early events (with explanations including absence of language or self-concept, or the fact that the key areas of our brain, e.g. the medial temporal lobes including the hippocampus, are very much under-developed at such an age). However, I'm not definitely saying this is not the case! It's simply that I'm trained to be an empiricist, so I would be hesitant to confidently affirm anything more without objective verification.

Well, our semester is about to start (next week) so I'd better get on with finalizing my lectures . . .

Best wishes,
Richard

One morning during the week before Christmas, five weeks after my stroke, the physiatrist came to see me during his rounds for
what I assumed was one of my periodic checkups. He may have
visited me as often as twice weekly. Nevertheless, for five weeks I
had the impression that he was monitoring my progress fairly closely,
although when I pestered him with questions about my prognosis
he rarely said anything, either encouraging or discouraging. He
would shrug his shoulders and say, "I don't know, I've never had a
stroke." It seemed to me that for a specialist he was disturbingly
mute on the subject of stroke in general and my recovery in particular. Later I would come to appreciate his candor.

"We're wondering if you would like to go home for Christmas?"
he asked. "And if things work out, return in the New Year as an
out-patient for three months. This would mean coming into the
hospital for five hours, four to five times a week."

I was both elated and a bit scared at the prospect. Wasn't he again
rushing things? Initially they had told me I would be a resident in
rehab for at least two months. What had changed?

For my part, I was fairly pleased with my recovery. I was now
able to stand on my own as long as I knew there was something or
someone nearby to break my fall. And I had started to climb the
stairs with the lowest rise on the stair platform. This was a structure
with four sets of stairs, each with a different rise, leading to a small
six-by-six-foot platform at the top. The top was no higher than five
normal stairs in height, not exactly K2 but a challenge nonetheless
to someone with a severe case of vertigo who was just learning to
walk again. With a railing to clutch onto and with a therapist holding on tightly to a "security" belt wrapped around my waist, I had
made it up three stairs before my legs buckled and I wanted to return to earth and the safety of my wheelchair.

I could also pedal the stationary bike for ten to fifteen minutes
without interruption before I felt winded and longed for a nap. And
lately, with the aid of a bed bar, I could pull myself into a sitting
position. This hurt if I didn't get my right side aligned properly and

if I got tangled up. Such episodes invariably ended with me franti-
cally pressing the buzzer and a nurse running to my assistance. I still
couldn't roll onto my left side, because my right side didn't want to
go with me, especially my right arm. When I finally learned to
make this manoeuvre several months later, I would grab my right
arm in my left hand and pull it with me when I twisted my body. I
used my left leg to lever my right leg forward and over when I
started the roll. Timing for this procedure was critical, like doing a
tumble run in gymnastics. And I still slept with pillows propping
me up, otherwise I tended to fall over or flop about like a landed
fish, especially when my leg or arm went into spasms.

Perhaps my greatest concern was that I definitely needed someone to help me get dressed and go to the bathroom. I could transfer
myself to the toilet without assistance, but I couldn't wipe myself. I
was still in my toddler phase. By this time in rehab my remaining
sense of modesty/timidity/shyness had evaporated. Any sense of exaggerated vanity had deserted me. Most of the time my dependency
on the nursing staff was comically absurd; I rang for their help with
irrational glee, but occasionally I felt a nagging frustration and an
unbearable sadness at my helplessness, such as a circus bear must feel
when trained to ride a bike.

All in all, though, I was making progress. My right leg now
moved, as did my right arm, up to a point. Most of the time my
right arm was fixed in one position, bent at the elbow at a ninety-
degree angle across my lower chest. For some reason I recalled a
portrait of Napoleon. And my fingers were frozen into a claw. But I
had a little movement in a couple of fingers, which I took to be a
positive sign, and my left hand had assumed many of the responsi-
bilities traditionally done by my right hand.

I hesitated, wondering why they wanted to make this change to
my original timetable for rehab. Were they trying to get rid of me?
Had I offended someone? My thoughts took flight as paranoia took
hold.

Then I panicked.

"Who'll take care of me?" I asked.

"Pat," he said and then he smiled. "Your wife? You do remember her, don't you?" He was trying to be funny, but I was terrified.

"Yes," I answered curtly.

Now he was pissing me off.

"We'll do a trial run over the weekend to see how Pat copes. If it's too much for her — and it will be demanding — then we'll return to our original plan. We just think you might manage better at home. You might find sleeping in your own bed preferable to sharing sleeping quarters with three other men." His hand made a sweeping gesture taking in the room. "Especially over the holiday when this place essentially shuts down. There'll be no therapy for that week anyway. Few of the regular staff will be around. Also, we've discovered that most people recover more quickly at home, in a familiar environment. In the meantime, we'll keep your bed on hold. Just in case. But if Pat's up to being a full-time caregiver, which we think she is, this change might speed up your recovery. What do you think?"

I didn't know what to think. Why the sudden rush?

Most of the nursing staff was attentive, compassionate and caring; I had grown used to their habits and peculiarities. And by now they knew what I needed when I had an emergency that required immediate attention. How would Pat manage me if I took a tumble or I shit myself? Would she tire of dressing me every day?

Occasionally visitors to other patients on the ward, who were often nervous, got under my skin. They didn't want to be there but felt some sort of obligation to visit an old friend. Whether or not they viewed their friends with sympathy I had no idea, but they saw the rest of us as aberrations. As a freak show. Was that how people were going to look at me on the outside? I wasn't sure I was ready for the glares of fear and disgust. And yet it would be a relief to be off the ward and living at home, as long as Pat could keep up with my considerable demands and needs. There were still so many things I couldn't do for myself. And my wheelchair was a major presence. It was like having a useful best friend move in who was constantly under foot.

But when I thought about it, I definitely wanted to go home and sleep in my own bed. I was a handful, yes. All of us were, on the ward, with our hallucinations, our erratic mood swings, our unpredictability. Our bewilderment. But home is where I belonged. I knew that.

"We'll supply all your medications for the weekend and we've given Pat requisitions to take to the Red Cross who will temporarily provide you with all the aids you need. Your own wheelchair, a walker, bed bar, bathing bench, commode, anything you think might make your home stay more comfortable."

Okay, I thought, being home was the best choice. Better food, less regimen, Pat for company. And home would be quiet and would give me time to think. I would finally be able to escape the persistent hum of the hospital, droning on and on like a hive of bees with its busy work.

"Well?"

He hesitated, studying me, his eyes trying to tug me back into the routine of daily life.

"If it's any comfort, we think you're ready. Pat's keen to give the idea a go. Enthusiastic support like hers is half the battle."

For a split second I didn't know how to answer.

"Yes," I said finally, rubbing my eyes which had become bleary, "if you think it's best."

"Good. I do. Wise decision."

As the physiatrist reached the door, he turned his head, smiled and said, almost as if an afterthought: "Merry Christmas."

Suddenly I felt euphoric. "Same to you," I answered, bemused. For a moment, I'd forgotten, completely forgotten, the time of year.

Home. Back in the real world. Home was definitely where I belonged.

Merry Christmas.

Home, Therapy
and Forest Bathing

Just after noon on Friday, Pat and Gerry James came to pick me up at the hospital for my trial weekend at home. (Gerry is a neighbour and friend, a former NHL and CFL hockey and football player about whom I'd written a book entitled *Kid Dynamite*, published in 2011, a biography based on his sports career.) At home I would be surrounded by a world of familiar objects, presumably aids to my recovery: books, paintings (my favourite called "Dickie" by my friend Ian Garrioch, a circular acrylic painting of a crow perched on a branch set against a night sky and the universe, one blue-green eye holding the viewer in its trance, as if inviting you to look through a hole or telescope out into space), an old lamp and chair (its curves and stuffing easy on the body), old carpets (one depicting the "Tree of Life"), a fireplace, a jade tree, dried flowers, pottery, and a stained glass window showing a heron standing before a blood-red sun and with leaded Chinese characters running down one side that read, when translated, "To know the dawn is to have it in your heart."

Sentimental, yes, but offering tenderness and comfort. Plus intimacy. Pat, I knew, would provide surety with her love.

A group of nurses and therapists had gathered at the car to see if I would be able to make the transfer from my wheelchair to the car seat without collapsing into a heap on the pavement. I think I surprised everybody, myself included. When I managed to stand, like a tin soldier, using the door and roof and my good left arm to help prop me up, I thought they were all going to applaud. Then I bent and folded back into the seat, and someone lifted my legs and feet after me into the car and fastened the seatbelt. I was ready to go, tucked in, like a Formula 1 driver. Speed at last, I thought; I looked forward to zipping through the traffic, escaping my confinement as if negotiating the final lap through the streets of Monaco.

Two things stood out in my mind as we made that forty-odd-kilometre road trip home.

Simple pleasures.

On our way along the Island Highway, we swung down onto an area of flatland that hugged the shores of Nanoose Bay, purportedly the deepest bay on the Pacific coastlines of both North and South America. Catching my first peek at the water, then the decaying posts of the old docks, the mussel and oyster farms, the moorage buoys for the larger naval ships that often visited the bay — in 1988, the USS *Missouri*, by this time a rusty old bucket of bolts, on its final voyage around the globe, had once spent a summer night anchored in the bay — I felt the sort of exhilaration and relief that some men feel after they've taken their first lover. Or the excitement one feels after the birth of a child. A moment of uncertainty followed by unqualified bliss.

One morning, several years earlier, when I still lived in a house by the edge of the sea, I remembered I had wakened at sunrise to a low grinding sound, like the sound made by the slower drill a dentist uses to carve out larger areas of tooth decay. My initial thought as I staggered out of bed was that the ocean was tearing away the huge riprap seawall in front of the house. I expected any minute the house would be washed out to sea. But what I saw when I reached the front porch was the longest tug I had ever seen, towing the *Ocean Ranger*, at that time rumoured to be the largest offshore oil rig in the world. It was gigantic, blocking from sight the islands that formed an archipelago at the mouth of the bay. Apparently Nanoose Bay was the perfect place to do a refit before they towed the monster rig around the tip of South America — it was too big to pass through the Panama Canal — to the oilfields off Newfoundland. Tragically, two years later, eighty-four men lost their lives when the rig sank after a rogue wave hit it during a winter storm. I think someone had left a hatch or window open.

Why did I remember these things?

The refit in the bay had to have happened in 1980 because Pat's dad, Tom, had been alive at the time. A retired welder and pipeliner, he and I launched his small fourteen-foot aluminum boat and ran out to survey the work being done on the thirty-storey rig. As he stared up into the bright-blue August sky, Tom shook his head and marvelled at the idea that oil could be extracted from below the seabed.

"It'll be a problem, though," he said, "the two don't mix. Oil and water. You know what they say."

A movie could have been made based on Tom's life, a hard but happy life. Two months before he died, Tom came to me and rather sheepishly asked if he should be worried that he was peeing blood. Foolishly I had lectured him about taking care of himself. At the time I was furious; I knew the effect this news would have on his family. Two weeks later his mother died, accidentally, after slipping on her way to the shower and breaking a hip. She was 101. Six weeks after that Tom followed her, at sixty-four. I still remember his huge, calloused hands as they fumbled with the cribbage pegs, and I could still hear his throaty laugh as he bellowed "deal."

As we drew closer to home, memories of the bay danced in my thoughts.

Summer evenings spent fishing off Maude Island, lounging in the warm water of tidal pools, hunting for the perfect shell with my daughter, playing catch with my son on a sandbar, carefree moonlit walks with Pat across miles of sand at low tide.

Simple pleasures.

Even though it was a cold December day, I had the passenger window of the car rolled down halfway so that I could breathe in the salty air. At low tide it had a pungent smell, a smell I loved, the smell of rot and rebirth. Pat and Gerry were both shivering, complaining that they were freezing, and with more patience than I likely deserved were insisting I close the window. But I gloried in the closeness of the cold sea and, as we sped along the highway, I leaned my forehead against the cool of the window and looked out past the bony trees, mostly maple, at the grey sea, so calm for the moment, like a polished sheet of metal. In the distance the mainland coastal mountains rose under a heavy layer of woolly-looking cloud, a softer grey than the sea, but all too sombre for my mood. In another three months the herring would return and all the sea grasses would be covered in roe.

Once again my senses seemed to be amplified, and for the first time since the stroke I felt joy. Everything had a clarity to it — perhaps nakedness is more apt — that I had never experienced before.

When we lost sight of the bay I fell asleep and didn't wake until we slowed down and pulled into our driveway. Again the trees stood out, especially the twisting shapes of the arbutus with their peeling bark and reddish flesh, like dancers caught momentarily in a pose, their proposition one of movement, slow and graceful.

The second thing that brought me much pleasure occurred when Gerry pushed me over the threshold of Pat's and my new home, a timber-frame house my brother Brian had designed and, with my brother Guy, had helped build. In that moment I understood the beauty of Brian's work. It was stunning, absolutely stunning; it had all the intricacies of a finely woven tapestry. Before this I hadn't fully appreciated his craftsmanship and vision. What struck me now was how alive each timber seemed, how organic the design felt. I could feel the energy it radiated.

Every timber glowed as if still running with sap; as if surrounded by an aura; as if existing in another dimension.

I sat in my wheelchair and stared up at the rafters and massive fir beams criss-crossing from one side of the house to the other. The symmetry, including the occasional odd angle, was exquisite, reminiscent of the ways in which constellations assumed the shapes of our imaginings and dreams. I remembered the engineer coming to the site during construction and saying, "I know it works mathematically, I know it's much stronger than it needs to be, but I don't know how your brother does it. I'm always amazed when I see the building lifted off the plans, the timbers in place like a sculpture, and then find myself walking inside the space that a short time ago was nothing but lines on sheets of paper."

And yet wasn't this the point, I wanted to ask him? To place yourself in a working relationship between the imaginative and the functional. The urge to create such a space was both intuitive and fundamental. And, without doubt, contemplative.

Directly above me a "taiko" beam spanned the distance between one exterior wall and a stately timber standing at the heart of the house. This "taiko" beam retained the original shape of its tree. In a Japanese home, such a beam would be given a prominent place in the structure, as a tribute to the forest. After all, trees had been holding up houses and defining the spaces they contained for as long as people had imagined hearth and home. Even though the forest could be a scary place, especially for kids who read stories such as the Brothers Grimm's *Hansel and Gretel*, trees had always comforted me with their quiet whispers.

But what surprised me most as I looked around the large open space, from kitchen to dining room to living room, was a sense of movement. Everything was engaged in a grand ballet, all the tawny beams pulsating with life, creating an intimacy the hospital lacked and I now longed for. At first I thought my eyes and brain were playing tricks on me. Why did everything appear to have an extra dimension to it? An extra clarity? Around each beam I could see a golden glow, and an absence of hard edges.

As I continued to look around the room from my wheelchair, none of the rules that had once defined reality for me held up. They were someone else's rigid and uncompromising constructs. As far as I could see, everything flowed into everything else. Everything was in continual flux. This convergence of things felt natural, although they were continually changing and redefining my relationship with them. What I saw was beautiful, not at all complex, not at all urgent, as I would have imagined. And while this gift of a new way of seeing gave me great pleasure, I began to worry.

If I told anyone what I was seeing I was certain they would think me crazy.

At once I clung to the winter rose Pat had cut from our neighbour's garden, a yellow flower with wilting brownish petals, which she had placed in a vase.

What had become of reality as I understood it?

And how was I present in this newly perceived reality?

I found then and still find now, two years later, that it's difficult to describe the way things appeared or sounded in those first months after my stroke. When I looked at a branch on a fir tree every individual needle stood out as if demanding my attention. "We're as important as the entire tree," they seemed to be saying. "Look at us if you want to see the whole." And my hearing for several months was off the charts. When Pat and I went for a walk, birds chirping in a blackberry thicket sounded like church bells ringing. My head the clapper.

Pat would ask, "What birds?"

I would stop walking, look up from my walker and suggest she get her hearing checked. "You're kidding, you must be going deaf."

A few months after my release as an out-patient, my friend Joe Rosenblatt sent me the link to an article that had recently run in the *Toronto Star* on July 30, 2013. The headline read, "Stroke rewires Toronto patient's brain so he 'feels' and 'tastes' colour." The byline went on to say: "St. Michael's Hospital researchers diagnose an extremely rare case of 'synesthesia' — only the second ever caused by a brain injury."

> The first time he felt like he could "ride" music he worried that something was seriously wrong.
>
> It was August 2008 and the patient, now in his mid-40s, had recently suffered a stroke. He was in his Toronto condo watching the opening ceremonies of the Beijing Olympics when, suddenly, the high-pitched falsetto of the opera singers sent him on a journey.
>
> "I felt myself get sucked into the TV set, transported through the wires, and wind up floating above the Olympic Stadium in Beijing," he told the *Star*. "It was such a real experience. I could feel the heat and humidity on my skin."
>
> He was not transported to Beijing that day. But as he would soon learn, the feeling he experienced was very real. He had acquired synesthesia, a rare condition that triggers more than one sense at the same time.
>
> Most often present at birth (famous synesthetes include singer-songwriter Billy Joel and painter Wassily Kandinsky), the condition is marked by unusual connections in the thalamus region of the brain. The result is a peculiar combination of senses: a letter of the alphabet can elicit colour; a specific sound, meanwhile, can prompt a smell.
>
> According to researchers at St. Michael's Hospital, who detailed the Toronto patient's case in the August issue of *Neurology*, his is the second-known instance of a person developing synesthesia as a result of a brain injury.

His condition came as a surprise to researchers at St. Michael's, where he was treated following his stroke. Although doctors quickly recognized his symptoms as synesthesia, they hadn't realized that the condition could be prompted by a brain injury, said study author and neuroscientist Tom Schweizer.

Upon scouring the literature, they found the only other reported case, a woman in the U.S. who, after having a stroke, felt a tingling sensation when she heard a certain tone.

But the synesthesia in their patient, who tasted blue when he ate raspberries, appeared to be much more profound, even linking emotions to colours and sounds.

In their study, Schweizer and his team focused on the patient's response to the James Bond movie theme song, which the patient described as sending him on "a ride that was cosmic in its voyage."

To see what happened in the brain in these moments, they put the patient in a functional MRI, which shows the areas of the brain involved in performing a given task. Upon hearing the high-pitched brass in the song, "huge areas of the brain lit up," Schweizer said.

Schweizer believes that when the patient recovered from his stroke, which occurred in the thalamus, the brain's central relay station, the wiring got "mixed," and linked "areas that wouldn't normally be in direct communication."

There is no treatment for synesthesia. But whereas those who are born with the condition can't control it, this patient "is able to turn it off and on, and can enjoy riding the wave," Schweizer said. "It's a good trip."

Despite the lingering physical challenges he faces, the patient said that if he were offered a pill that could erase all the effects of his stroke, he would decline.

As is so often the case these days when reporting the news, the claim the reporter made that this was only the second case "ever" of brain injury causing synesthesia seemed a bit of an exaggeration.

How could anyone possibly know it was only the "second" case? I'm sure, if asked — and herein lies the rub, no one asks — many stroke survivors would be able to recount stories about changes to their perceptions, some fantastical if not unbelievable. But they remain silent for fear of censure. Because such experiences aren't within the realm of the interlocutor's experience, the stroke patient is told he's either crazy or mistaken or imagining things, things that can't be statistically proven and therefore don't exist. This quarrel aside, I found the article intriguing. Perhaps, I hoped, this case explained in part what had been happening inside my own brain and to my senses.

As Professor J. Allan Hobson of the Harvard Medical School argues in a brief but provocative "first-person account" of the stroke he suffered while travelling in Europe in February of 2001, "Consciousness can be studied only if subjective experience is documented and quantified, yet first-person accounts of the effects of brain injury on conscious experience are as rare as they are potentially useful."

While I don't claim to have experienced synesthesia, I do know that for several months after my stroke I saw and heard things differently. I have used the word "amplified" — augmented, deepened, heightened, intensified, all would work as well — but there is a point at which words no longer make sense, when the conjunction of things embodies a mystery that has been present since the beginning of time.

And in the face of that mystery we find a way to tell story.

Why else write, paint, sculpt, sing, dance, act out?

On a practical level, our house was ideal for someone in a wheelchair.

When drawing up the house plans, Brian had insisted that every door in the house be thirty-six inches wide.

"Just in case," he said.

"Just in case of what?" we asked.

"You never know," he answered, "what might happen. Things sneak up on you. Happen unexpectedly. You might as well be prepared."

And Brian knew all too well the vagaries of chance. What others might have called karma. He had lost an eye to what had been diagnosed as a harmless basal cell cancer on his cheek. When they followed what was supposed to have been a simple trail to the root of a minor problem, it led to a large tumour behind his eye.

He had been right. You never knew.

Now his comment seemed prophetic, his worry becoming a reality far earlier than either Pat or I had expected.

I remembered how upset one of the amputees at the hospital had been when the occupational therapist went to assess his home and returned with the news that he would have to remove all the doors in his house. At thirty inches wide, a wheelchair could just barely squeeze through the opening, but only if there was no door!

"How am I supposed to live in a doorless house?" he stammered. "What about privacy?"

Indeed, what about privacy, I wondered? As far as I knew, there were only two of them living in their small apartment. In their eighties what could they conceivably have to hide from one another? What happened behind closed doors? Perhaps that's where he searched through his diary of memories. Flipping pages in his mind. And he needed to be alone to do so. Or perhaps he removed his hearing aids and listened to the silence from a time before he was born and had married the woman he still loved. Surviving a stroke or the amputation of a limb makes you no less of a human being; you retain the same desires and feelings of grief with which you were born.

We all need our moments alone. But for most of the world a private space is a luxury few can afford. I remembered how Galsan Tschinag, a Tuvan writer from Mongolia whose first novel, *The*

Blue Sky, I had published in an English translation in 2006, had described life in a yurt. Inside the felt skin made of sheep's wool was an open space shared by an entire family, including livestock and pets. In that harsh landscape, outdoors, between the earth and the sky, was where you found a place to be solitary with your thoughts.

And as far as I knew, there would be no place for a wheelchair on the steppes of the high Altai Mountains.

Brian had also talked us into polished concrete floors throughout the house, with in-floor heating. At the time we had wondered if we could live with "the look," something akin to putting down grey granite everywhere.

"It's durable, like marble, and easy to keep clean," he had said. And then added, "Besides, they look good."

But now appearances had become a secondary concern. As Gerry inched me into the room I realized how easy it was going to be to wheel around the house. I would need to take a run at a couple of the rugs to get the wheelchair over the lip; otherwise getting from room to room was going to be a breeze. A smooth ride. And the kitchen bar, at chest height, would be ideal to lean on and do my exercises. Squats and step-overs; balancing on one leg; toe and heel rises, with both feet; arm and finger flexes. Little repetitive exercises for a body confined to a wheelchair and just beginning to relearn basic movements.

As I sat there and surveyed the rooms, Gerry became increasingly antsy. At seventy-eight he had not yet learned how to be still. He jumped about like someone roasting and selling chestnuts on a busy London street corner on an icy winter's night. As much as I was grateful for his help, I wanted him to leave. He was making me anxious.

Besides, since waking earlier that morning, I had been concentrating on one thing: getting home and taking a shower. In the hospital, weekly bathing had been a great relief but too hasty and robotic. This was no one's fault, but the experience had been more like being run through a car wash than taking the leisurely soak I was used to. You got slathered with soap and hosed down from nose to bumper. Everything had to be done according to a timetable drawn up in some remote administrative corner of the hospital.

And I felt, if not smelled, "ripe."

Finally I said, "Go, Gerry, you've been a great help. Now I need to sleep."

Sleep had become my "default" excuse when I wanted to be left alone.

"You're sure you'll be all right?"

"Yes, we'll be fine," Pat said, as she ushered him towards the door.

"Okay, okay, I know when I'm not wanted," he whined, feigning the appearance of someone caught between disdain and hurt. His face scrunched up into a pout.

In spite of his gentle protest I could see that he was relieved to be leaving. What's important to understand here is how vital people like Gerry were to my recovery. I was thankful for his empathy and willingness to help. Pat could bear only so much of the worry and the load of minute-to-minute care. And Gerry, along with other friends, helped to lessen the burden I feared I'd already become.

Stroke survivors often develop feelings of guilt. A painful sense of inadequacy begins to eat away at whatever confidence has survived. No longer able to fend for themselves, their dependency on others becomes corrosive. To compound this pervasive sense of insecurity, a UK study, reported in the *Daily Mail* on October 8, 2014, indicated that 50 percent of stroke survivors feel abandoned when released from hospital.

Another friend, Keith Harrison, an old colleague from my teaching days, forwarded for several months each issue of his subscription to *The New York Review of Books*. It didn't matter that at first I couldn't lift the paper to read it; what mattered was the contact from an old friend and the feeling that he still considered me a part of the world to which I'd once belonged.

Rabbit has brain, each issue proclaimed!

Perhaps the most convenient feature Brian had incorporated into the house design was a "wet room" in the ensuite bathroom, essentially a shower without doors or a ledge separating it from the rest of the room. It had three different shower heads which I could easily access from a seated position on the mobile commode Pat had borrowed from the Red Cross. Once undressed, a major job in itself, I could roll into the wet room and soak to my heart's content. Letting the water cascade over my head and down my body seemed the pinnacle of satisfaction and well-being.

My God, I reflected, my life has become a series of ridiculously simple pleasures. I've become as soft as a ripened peach. But I'm still alive. What was "me" before the stroke still lies beneath my skin, still flourishes in my mind. I could feel it then, and over the next two years it would grow to become the self I am now.

Over the weekend I had showered twice, watched some television — the news hadn't changed, things were as bizarre and as absurd as ever — and slept. To my surprise, watching television made me feel dizzy. The picture jerked about in a busy and disconnected way and no matter where we set the volume it seemed too loud. And if there were plots to some of the dramas we watched, I couldn't follow them. At one point I had rolled into my study to look longingly at book spines and titles. I desperately wanted to read again, but I still couldn't hold a book in one hand and open it with the other. It weighed too much. Nor could I turn pages. My right arm either hung limply at my side or, more likely, continued to suffer from painful spasms, a form of hyperflexion, and still flexed into a rigid right angle which I held across my chest. My hand formed into a tight little fist and refused to open.

Uninterrupted sleep gave me the most pleasure, especially knowing that Pat was nearby — so that's what I did: sleep, through most of those two days and three nights. In the few days I had available to plan this adventure from my hospital bed, I don't know what it was

I conjured up; I think it probably included erotic fantasies of some sort, but whatever it was I imagined, the reality was a long "snore." Literally. Even in my wheelchair I nodded off, my chin pushing forward and resting on my chest.

Pat set up a bedside table on which she placed my new urinal and anything else I might need. She had also borrowed a bed bar from the Red Cross. If I needed to get out of bed to go to the bathroom I could pivot myself into a sitting position, find my walker and shuffle to the toilet. While the distance was short, the feeling of accomplishment was great. To be free of the wheelchair was incredibly liberating. I felt almost human. I was a biped once again, although the length of time I was able to support myself in a standing position was depressingly brief. My right leg still tagged along after me like an orphaned animal. And sometimes, when the contractions occurred, both my leg and foot performed an odd tap dance; they seemed to have lives of their own.

Soon my sense of euphoria was punctured. While I had figured out how to pull on my shirt and pants, wash my face and brush my teeth with my left hand — with the occasional bashing and bleeding of my gums — I couldn't reach my rear end or my feet. Wiping myself and putting on my socks and shoes were beyond me. I needed help and had to call Pat for assistance.

Dressing was like trying to escape from a straitjacket, in reverse.

When I looked down at my shoelaces, I realized I couldn't even tie a simple bow!

Again I wanted to weep. I felt so helpless and useless.

And when the old weariness and despair set in, I slipped sideways, plunging aimlessly off the edge of any known map of the world. My tongue thickened and my speech once again became slurred and incoherent.

I began to wonder how much of my dependency Pat could take. When would she reach a reasonable, a tolerable limit? I worried she would become frustrated and eventually overwhelmed by my constant hounding, by my impotence, by my odious-repulsive-monstrous being, but over that first weekend — and in the months that followed — she never wavered from her determination and belief that I was going to make a full recovery.

What a blessing this encouragement was for me — this faith which surrounded her like a magical cloak.

Early Monday morning we drove slowly back into the hospital, both Pat and I reliving and relishing the last two days we had spent together. Alone. At home. Now we were being sucked back into the bureaucracy, some jokester's clever idea of order and efficiency. I wanted something far more clandestine. Like poaching the laird's trout or pheasant or prized stag.

The trial weekend had been a success, but I had to return to the rehab unit to be formally released. I couldn't simply fade away or run for it, which would have proven me ungrateful, which I wasn't. I had to be discharged through the proper channels; otherwise I might be declared AWOL. There would be papers to sign, instructions and medications to pick up, schedules to follow. I was about to become an out-patient expected to follow a specific and demanding daily routine.

My life was going to be organized into little segments devoted to my recovery as well as to my reintegration into society, back into the "real" world. And what an odd world it was, as far as I could see.

After we had parked the car in the handicap zone in front of the rehab unit and Pat had fetched my wheelchair from the trunk, I was seized by panic. What if my trial homestay had failed in the eyes of the physiatrist? But that was a silly worry. How would he or anyone else know whether or not my short furlough had been a success? As I hauled myself into an upright position to transfer to my wheelchair I looked at the brick facade with its bank of blank windows. Each window reflected a scene of the parking lot, a busy intersection, the apartment buildings beyond and the intricate old Japanese cherry tree woven into the sky that I'd spent so many hours studying and that in some odd way had become a talisman for me. I fancied that when it blossomed pink in early spring, I would once again walk.

Behind each reflection were minds and bodies in various stages of disrepair. As far as I knew, patients rarely looked out at the passing world. Such daring might be construed as an invitation promising hope, and such anticipation was too often fraught with disappointment. I realized then how much I dreaded returning to this place, in spite of the wonderful care I had received. Long ago I had stopped casting myself as the beleaguered inmate in some terrible prison drama and had come to understand that my keepers did their utmost to ease my pain and inspire recovery. They were good-hearted people. And yet, as fond as I was of most of them, I didn't want to return to the hospital, not as a resident. It would be fine to come back each day for a few hours of therapy. I could see the benefit in that, but the prospect of checking back in, of reclaiming my bed, was unthinkable. To be assaulted by the smells and sounds and sights of a ward fighting to postpone the devastation of atrophy would be a form of torture, especially after the weekend of peace and quiet optimism I had experienced at home. I had tasted the possibility of a new life, of what I now saw as a potential rebirth.

This raised the important question, though: Where did I belong?

And how much say would I have in where I spent my immediate future?

Our first meeting to discuss my out-patient status was in my old room at 10:00 a.m. with Elvira, the head nurse, from the rehabilitation unit. Jack, the "Bird Man," watched, his face beaming, pleased for me, I thought, while Pat collected my few remaining things. Extra shirts, pants, socks, underwear, my shaving kit, which I hadn't used in weeks. My beard had grown in white and made me look like Santa Claus. The two amputees were probably in the gym doing therapy.

Her name reminded me of *Elvira Madigan*, the title of a stylish and beautiful Swedish film from the 1960s which used the second movement of Mozart's 21st piano concerto as its theme. The concerto was one of my favourite pieces of music, and the film, shot from unconventional points of view, the camera always retreating, fading away, was an improbable romance based on a true story. A young tightrope walker falls in love with a Swedish cavalry officer fourteen years her senior. Today the site in Denmark of their consensual suicide is marked by a white stone that attracts lovers and tourists from all over the world. Until that moment, until she introduced herself, I hadn't thought of or heard the name Elvira in fifty years.

"How was your weekend?" she asked. "You must be honest with me if we're to make a constructive assessment of which therapy would be best for you."

I thought I could hear the trace of a German accent, but before I could ask she volunteered an answer.

"Austrian," she said, clearly anticipating my question. I felt embarrassed. How could I be so brazen? "Many years ago," she added.

"Fine," I said, "the weekend was fine. Everything went surprisingly well. I even managed to walk from the bed to the toilet before I needed to call for help."

Why was I trying to be clever? Boastful? Ironic?

And then, as if I couldn't be trusted, Elvira and I turned to look at Pat.

"Yes, it went very well," Pat said.

"You didn't have any problems?"

"Not really. He wants to be more independent than he is."

"Of course, that's natural. Especially with someone so determined." She smiled at me as if to tell me she understood my impertinence. "Have you any questions?"

"Does this mean I'm free to go?" I asked.

"Yes, if you think you're ready and Pat agrees. The decision is really for the two of you to make. Let me say, experience shows that recovery happens much more quickly in the comfort of your own home. I'm sure the doctor explained all this when he suggested you become an out-patient. The most important thing is that you both feel confident in each other. You mustn't try the impossible or be too demanding, and Pat must feel that she's equal to the task."

For me the answer was simple. I preferred to be at home in Pat's care as long as she didn't mind responding to my almost hourly needs, which could be not only demanding but, well, at times, gross. From rolling me over to cleaning me. In many respects it would be like caring for an infant again. When we had discussed my becoming an out-patient, I tried to be as graphic as possible. Perhaps exaggerating details, although I don't think so. No rosy pictures. Pat had shrugged and said, "Remember? The small church, St. Francis-in-the-Wood? For better or worse."

"And there will also be the driving," I added. "A lot of driving. At least four days a week. Between home and the hospital. Most days I'll be in therapy for four to five hours, over lunch. That could become very tedious."

She had squeezed my limp, unresponsive hand and said, "We'll do this. Together." And then, briefly, from a silent place of strength and endurance, she took control. The decision was made.

"Before we finalize everything," I said, glancing up from my wheelchair at Elvira, suddenly conscious of a nagging uneasiness, "I have a couple of questions. Concerns."

"Shoot," she said. She loved colloquialisms, her favourite being "far out," another reminder of the sixties.

"Will there be someone around to monitor my vitals? Like my blood pressure and blood sugar?"

"Yes," she said, grinning, "me."

"Who will be my doctor?"

"Your GP, except when you're in the hospital. And then you'll be under the supervision of one of the physiatrists or hospitalists. Don't worry, we've got you covered."

"And if I have an emergency — say I have to use the bathroom and Pat isn't here — will there be someone willing to help me?"

Finally, I was admitting what was at the crux of my unease. Fifty years later and I was still the young man staring down at the floor in the public washroom in Paris. What strange cargoes we carry around with us, sometimes for our entire lives.

"Yes," Elvira said, "anyone on the team will be able and willing to help."

And just as suddenly I realized my release had been a mere formality, probably had been from the minute I left my room on Friday.

Subject, of course, to Pat's approval.

Certain rituals have an order and pace to them that never varies.

Elvira arranged a meeting for shortly after lunch with my rehab team: members included Elvira herself who was the team leader; Deb, a physiotherapist; Barb, an occupational therapist; and Tina, a social worker. Later, Helena was added as an assistant to the two therapists. This was the dedicated and conscientious little troupe that hoped to guide me back to the world of the "living."

We sat squeezed around a table in a small office next to the gym. Elvira introduced everyone and explained their roles in my rehabilitation. Over the Christmas break I would likely have a couple of light workout sessions, but rigorous therapy wouldn't begin in earnest until the new year. 2013. The number kept climbing, signalling the end of my seventieth year. A few weeks ago I wasn't even sure I would get to the new year. This would be a wonderful opportunity to catch up on some much-needed rest, she said. They all knew how demanding and stressful prolonged confinement in hospital could be on the body and spirit.

Did they, I wondered, did they really know?

And did they know what was going on in my mind?

Busily they all scribbled into notebooks as I answered questions about my stroke and commented on the progress I felt I'd made so far.

"First of all," I told them, "you can understand what I'm saying, can't you?"

They nodded and smiled.

"Well, that's one thing that's decidedly better," I said, "especially when I have something to say."

Right away I noticed I was slurring my words. I could hear myself, the slippery syllables sliding into one another like cartoon figures on ice. Anxiety had that effect on me.

Did they notice? Would I be rejected from the program before I'd even entered it?

I wanted to tell the team that I had stopped drooling and that I could now eat, but that was probably known or self-evident.

Then I blurted out, "I still have certain handicaps. There are things I can't do for myself and for which I need assistance, but then the wheelchair in which I'm sitting is probably a pretty good clue to those limitations."

I gasped. Had I really said that entire sentence without pause?

They laughed. Everyone was so cheerful. Perhaps it was the season.

The questions continued, ending with: What did I most hope to achieve through my rehabilitation? I answered in the way that I expected most stroke survivors would have answered, if they could have answered at all: I wanted to be normal. I wanted to return to the person I was prior to the stroke. They shook their heads, their eyes searching mine to see if I were joking or, more likely, if I were a misguided simpleton. They were right, of course, such a wish was folly. I knew it; they knew it. I remember thinking, I don't really know how to answer that question.

Besides, I had my own more urgent questions, two on which my sanity and well-being hinged. At least as far as I was concerned. Why was no one telling me what I really wanted to know: What had caused my stroke? And could it happen again?

No one, not a soul, had these answers.

After what seemed like an interminable silence, I said, "Walk."

Out of the blue, without coaxing, I repeated, "Walk," followed by a confused silence. Everyone looked at me blankly, as if I were conversing with myself. I looked around the circle, from face to face, trying to detect a simple sign that would reveal my fate. I couldn't get the timing right. We seemed to be speaking at cross-purposes.

"I suppose what I want most from rehab is to walk again," I said, hoping to pick up on a thread that had obviously been lost. "I have a dream that Pat and I will once again be able to stroll through the back streets of Rome or Paris, or through the parks of London or Geneva. Or along the forest paths at Cathedral Grove. Or over the sand and logs at Long Beach to stick a foot in the waters of the Pacific."

Had I known then what I know now, almost two years later, I would have said, "Move my fingers well enough to type or play the piano." I would have given this answer because I know now that if you can move your fingers and wiggle your toes, the rest of your limbs will have recovered. The nerves in the most distant extremities are the last to heal, are the last to reconnect with the brain.

Deb jotted something into her notebook; Barb grabbed her lower lip between her teeth and glanced from me to the floor, while Elvira and Tina smiled in a way intended to comfort me.

Obviously they had already talked amongst themselves. Everything, I realized, absolutely everything had been decided before Pat and I had even arrived at the hospital.

"Sometime in the next few weeks," Tina said, "a district nurse will be coming around to your home to see if she can offer any suggestions that might help make your lives easier."

Oh joy, I thought.

Christmas Eve. From my wheelchair I watched Pat decorate the Great Room: with lights hanging around the dining-room windows;

with cotton batting along the mantel above the gas fireplace on which she placed nativity scene figures; with a small lighted tree she and Nicole had made one Christmas with garlands of blue tinsel; with red and white candles stuck in brass holders; and with cuttings from the cedar and holly trees in the garden which she made into wreaths and table displays. Busy and fiddly work. Work to occupy the hands and mind. Of all the West Coast trees, cut cedar gives off a scent that fills the nostrils and imagination with a sense of bittersweet remorse. It reminds us of keepsakes and of warm, old sweaters stored in wooden chests. And perhaps asks the question, why have you forsaken me? Along the windowsill she stood cards, both those which had been sent to me over the last several weeks with well-wishes and those that contained season's greetings.

"We need a touch of the green," she said. "Something to cheer us up."

My memories of past Christmases were mixed. As a young boy I had sung soprano in a church choir. Dressed in our white cassocks, hair trimmed short, the boy's section of the choir was the perfect picture of innocence and health. Red-cheeked and full of voice. One year, when I was nine or ten, we had been featured live at Christmas on national radio, and when we got to my solo verse as the third king in the carol "We Three Kings of Orient Are" I forgot the lyrics:

> Myrrh is mine, its bitter perfume
> Breathes a life of gathering gloom;
> Sorrowing, sighing, bleeding, dying,
> Sealed in the stone-cold tomb.

For years after that humiliating moment, all the lyrics were seared into my memory. As I looked back on that day, I figured I had good reason to forget those words which chilled me with their ominous message. They said: everyone I loved was eventually going to die. I was going to die. What was "Merry" about the confluence of Christmas with the Crucifixion? I remember as I looked up at the Christ figure on the cross hanging above the altar, blood dripping from his palms and feet, I envisioned all sorts of cruel and unnecessary torture. Nothing could dress up and make sense of the Crucifixion, especially not the story of three wise men, probably Persian, following a distant star to the stable and manger in Bethlehem.

Then I had been one confused and cynical kid. Now I was one tired and bewildered older man — living inside a stroke.

As a parent I had received ample pleasure through the years from watching our kids unwrap Christmas presents. What frenzy. I was amazed by how fast meticulously wrapped parcels were turned into a free-for-all of paper, tape, ribbons and bows. My flesh and blood became whirling dervishes, noisy, confident, excited, filled with all the festive energy that was supposed to be powered by the belly laugh of old St. Nick. Ho, ho, ho. A snowfall on Christmas Eve added to the jubilation and mystique.

And yet, as I was growing up, Christmas and New Years were two days about which I felt ambivalent. In fact, the whole season had always filled me with both joy and sadness. Joy because that's when family and friends gathered to express and show their love for one another, when kinship truly seemed to matter. Sadness because rather than focusing my mind on birth and renewal, I tended to dwell on loss and time passing. "The stone-cold tomb" awaiting us.

Now I preferred to celebrate the winter solstice. A golden sunrise spreading across the snow-capped coastal mountains to the east and later a full moon rising out of the sea, passing across the night sky and illuminating the tidal flats. The days would be getting longer. The uninhabited, empty hours, shorter. I craved something simpler, more elemental. For that reason I had grown to love Stonehenge's and Avebury's mysteries. Those pagan circles presumably celebrating nature's cycle, days of rest following the harvest, days of preparation readying for the spring planting.

I was exhausted. From what I remember, Christmas Day, 2012,

passed in delicious sleep. There was nothing sinister in this, nothing symbolic. I had crawled out of bed, transferred to my wheelchair and joined Pat for breakfast. That was the full extent of my ambition. Within an hour, I had returned to bed.

I was looking forward to the arrival of Nicole, Iain and, most of all, our granddaughter, Flora, on Boxing Day. Christmas is for children and any form of celebration would have been incomplete without her. Like plum pudding without brandy. Pat had already begun to prepare a belated Christmas feast. I could hear her puttering in the kitchen and smell the baking — mince tarts and shortbread — as I fell asleep.

Rain beat against the "tin" roof and skylight, a soporific sound, not that my weariness needed help or accompaniment.

The next day, when the young family came through the front door, I saw Flora flinch and grab her mother's skirt. As soon as she saw me she frowned and nudged Nicole, the whole time keeping her eyes on me in case I might do something unexpected. Hesitantly she gave Pat a hug, never taking her gaze off of me. What had happened to Poppa? Why was he wearing this chair with large wheels? Was he like a jack-in-the-box? Would he suddenly spring at her? Or grow another head? In a week she would turn three, but at no age can you be prepared to see your "Poppa" folded into a wheelchair. As tearful as I felt, I could understand why the chair was an obstacle to any sort of physical contact. Throughout the day and dinner, she chatted to me, yet always from a distance, as if my spirit, the "real" me, were ephemeral or a construct of her imagination. And so we talked, as if through the bars of a cage, or between different realms, her movements timid and tentative, her words inquisitive and tender.

She was intrigued by my wheelchair. And fearful.

"They're my legs," I told her, "until Poppa gets better."

The sorrow I felt at that moment choked me, and I'm certain that if my lips had parted, the whole neighbourhood would have sworn they'd heard a lone wolf cry in the wilderness.

As they were leaving the next morning, Flora said, "Poppa, please get better."

A year would pass before she felt confident enough to approach me and wrap her arms around my legs. What a moment that was to treasure and for which to be thankful. By then I was walking short distances with the assistance of a cane.

My memory of Christmas week is largely a blank file. Mostly I slept, without interruption, oh so peaceful, but for a couple of hours each day I would roll in my wheelchair to a window and look out on the trees, ponds and lush green fairways of the golf course adjacent to where we live. Our house is secluded, surrounded by arbutus, fir, balsam, hemlock, maple, alder and cedar trees. A few years back, a friend, visiting us from Italy, had said we lived in a tree house. Everywhere you look, Nicoletta had said, you look out onto a forest. Onto the tops of trees.

After lying for weeks in hospital, surrounded by curtains and by the perpetual machinery of health care, suddenly to be able to feast on the sights and sounds of the natural world inspired a kind of awe, restful and yet life-affirming. In a couple of months, nuthatches, sparrows, warblers, swallows, chickadees, towhees, red-winged blackbirds, finches, robins (who had nested the past two years on one of the roof timbers) and at least two pairs of northern flickers would return to the house and garden. I had been thrilled and worried for its survival when I saw a Rufous hummingbird visit one of the outdoor plants on the patio, probably looking for food. For the first time I could appreciate why birding had become a passion for two old friends, Kieran and Pattie Kealy, who had come to see me in my second week in hospital; and for Mike Yip, whose remarkable photographs caught the split-second action in which birds defined and claimed their place in the spatial continuum. By comparison our movements were clumsy. Wasn't this what we did when we judged gymnastic or skating competitions — assess our lack of elegance?

From my roost I watched the solitary mute swan, graceful and dishonoured, cruise the ponds, often taking his frustration out on the geese. For some reason he didn't mind the company of the wigeons, buffleheads, scoters and ducks; the Canada geese he stalked as if they were an invading army. A gaggle of storm troopers. The swan's wings had been clipped so that he couldn't fly and the management of the golf course had separated him from his mate because the stately birds were considered an invasive species and therefore — according to the Audubon Society — shouldn't be allowed to propagate. What cruel punishment, I thought, to sentence any creature, innocent of everything but being what it was, to live out its existence alone.

Even a pond bustling with life can be a prison.

In the first or second week of out-patient therapy, two old friends, Bill and Elaine Coleman, came from Vancouver to spend the day. They had been in touch with Pat soon after she had sent out her first email reporting my stroke. I had been an usher at their wedding in the mid-sixties after which they went to Taiwan where Bill completed four and a half years of graduate work in Chinese History and Mandarin. He was fluent in the language and had a reading knowledge of around five thousand characters. Impressive for any student of the language, let alone a foreigner, and yet, he had told me on one occasion, there were still texts he couldn't read. Elaine had taught ESL to Chinese students and part-time at the American School in Taipei.

Bill had gone on to have a successful career as a Sinologist, working for various trading organizations that did business throughout Asia. In 1979 he had set up the Canada-China Trade Council, subsequently renamed the Canada China Business Council. He now had his own small and successful trading company and continued to make yearly excursions into a broadening Asian market. From what I gathered, ice wine was one of his big sellers. He wrote to say that on a recent visit to Shanghai he had met a Professor An, a faculty member in English at one of the local universities. Bill had told An about my illustrated children's book, *Elf the Eagle,* and An immediately expressed interest in doing a Chinese translation. When Bill informed An about my stroke, An sent me the following note:

Dear Ron,

Jasmine is not happy these days. Two of her baby teeth started playing tricks on her when she wolfed down a bar of chocolate. Since then, her appetite has been disturbed from time to time. Her mother and she worried for a while, but I persuaded them successfully to be at ease by describing my funny and adventurous experience of fighting against a big bone with no front teeth when I was 8. New things always come to us no matter we are ready or not. Sorry to know that you are now fighting with the stroke, but please do not worry too much. I do believe the winter is just a warming up program for the spring.

Do you believe that a 72 year old guy still maintains six marvelous abdominal muscles? My friend Professor Li is the very person. He is the guy who knows the secret of happy life. Bill has also met him and talked with him for a while. He kindly gave four pieces of advice for your consideration.

1. If possible, move to places where you can be very close to woods. Oxygen there is quite good to persons of acid constitution. And find some time to touch the trunk of a big tree while walking around it. Big trees have certain positive energy to help purify our blood and body.

2. Take the shower nozzle close to the top of the head very frequently when have the hot shower.

3. Before go to bed, put feet into a basin full of hot water for about 5–10 minutes (the water should be a little bit hot) and massage the bottom of the feet for about 5 minutes after washing feet.

4. Go on a light diet and be happy all the time.

Really hope his advice can be useful and keep my fingers crossed for your quick recovery.

By the way, Ron, an electronic version of *Elf* will be wonderful for me! Attached please find photos of Jasmine, professor Li and I.

Keep in touch!

Yours,
An

What a surprisingly intimate email to receive from someone I had never met. I was flattered and somewhat perplexed by the reference to An's daughter, but seriously willing to take the advice Professor Li offered. Everything he advised made perfectly good sense to me. The photo An had attached of Professor Li showed a lithe man who appeared to be in his late forties, early fifties, not a man of seventy-two. Posed as he was, he looked more like a martial arts master than a professor of English. Obviously his simple rules for a healthy life had worked for him. Or was it a matter of optics and my willingness to believe that a new "me" was possible, even with the simplest of cures? Whatever the case, the diet part of his advice had taken care of itself while I had been in hospital — I had lost over forty pounds in eight weeks — and, aside from the infrequent morose spells, I figured I was fairly upbeat for someone who had recently suffered a stroke. The ups and downs continued, but with less frequency.

Footbaths were an almost-forgotten experience. An's email jogged my memory. As a boy I remembered taking a rare footbath, in a white enameled pan, but not as a cure for anything. And definitely not as a part of any regular routine. Possibly my mother had insisted on them for the chills, as a precaution, after I had spent a day playing outside in heavy winter weather, in rain or wet snow. And in the winds that blew in off the Fraser River and Salish Sea. My adoptive mother was constantly trying to keep illness at bay. When it came to my sister and me, she was very health conscious — perhaps one of her ways of expressing her maternal instincts.

When I asked Pat to read An's email, in particular the mention of footbaths, she said: "What a great idea. Maybe it'll help with the edema and pain." Both my right foot and hand were as badly swollen as ever. Then she fetched the basin in which she cooked the Christmas turkey, filled the basin with hot water and had me sit down on the side of the bed and stick my feet in it. A few minutes into the ritual she began to massage my feet with soap. What a wonderful sensation. I loved the pampering and right away felt the tension and pain ease from my body. I already knew that standing under the rain shower head had a powerful effect on my entire being, that it helped me relax. Now the combination of the footbath and shower reminded me of my previous life when I would soak in the bathtub, from head to toe, for ages, and embrace the water as if I had been freed into a new element. Which, of course, I had. I remembered that then not only did I feel less tense, I felt revitalized. Lighter.

But the piece of advice that intrigued me most was the first: "Move to places where you can be very close to woods. And find some time to touch the trunk of a big tree while walking around it." While I lived in a house situated in the midst of trees, I rarely interacted with them. At least not directly. Sometimes I was tempted to speak to them, discreetly, but I rarely did. I was afraid my neighbours might see or hear me, and such behaviour was certain to fire up the rumour mill.

And yet you never know for sure where therapy begins, or what will give it greater force.

Before my stroke, I had been an avid gardener, and as soon as I arrived home from hospital I spent many of my waking hours meditating "on" but not "in" the garden. From behind windows I watched the swaying of different trees, their branches moving like calligraphers' brushes writing against the sky. The idea, though, of actually walking in and around the trees and touching them, as a healing rite, hadn't occurred to me. Admittedly, I had always believed in the power of nature to heal, and I had always found walks through wooded areas reinvigorating. And certainly Native lore and stories supported such beliefs. So why, at this critical time in my life, hadn't I made the connection between the forest that surrounded me and my own rehabilitation?

A few weeks after out-patient therapy began, when I was finally able to move about in a limited way with my walker, I made a point of visiting the grove of thirty to forty trees at the front of our property at least once a day. Why I hadn't done this in my wheelchair I didn't know. And following Professor Li's advice, I made a habit of running my palms over the bark of the different trees. The skin of fir and cedar trees was rough; the arbutus, stripped naked, felt cool and smooth, like burnished metal. Each tree had its own way of speaking and gave off its own particular energy.

When I became more mobile, I extended my walks to the lane that runs the length of the property, a distance of about two hundred feet, under an arching canopy of budding maples, down to the ponds, a thriving frog habitat. Around the edges, bulrushes and yellow irises flourished in mud, and I imagined that in spring this would probably be where the frogs would lay their eggs, in amongst the roots. In a few weeks, as the setting sun neared the equinox, a chorus of thousands of little green and brown tree frogs would begin their evening mating song. What a splendid sound all that hormonal energy produced. I had read somewhere that ecosystems with such robust amphibian populations were supposed to be particularly healthy. I hoped this was the case.

Tree frogs seemed a little less cautious than other creatures, perhaps because they blend into their surroundings so well. Not only can they change colour, they are wonderful ventriloquists. They throw their voices, so that listeners will think they're somewhere else. All the same, as emboldened and as friendly as they are, I worried about their safety, especially when biologists kept reminding us that they are an endangered species. I had seen several of them climbing door jambs and the cedar shingles that clad our house, and I had heard a couple croak from within the aluminum railing that wound around the patio. They seemed to like the echo that bounced back to them. Perhaps this was a new way to fall in love with yourself: by responding to your own echo.

What I did know for certain is that I felt much better. I was now convinced that my recovery was linked to the happiness of frogs as well as to the serenity nurtured by trees.

Cynics might think me gullible, more likely a fool. Wasn't I stating the obvious? Who in their right mind would argue against the fact that "getting a breath of fresh air" was good for you? Such platitudes were just plain old common sense. Yet over the following weeks of out-patient therapy, I came to believe Professor Li's advice was helping with my recovery. It was, in fact, medicinal. I had absolutely no evidence for this claim except to say I felt better. I had relearned the benefits of "being" in the outdoors.

Several months later Pat told me about an episode she'd watched on TV on David Suzuki's *The Nature of Things* in which he followed research on the benefits of *Shinrin-Yoku*, or Japanese "forest bathing." According to recent Japanese research, discussed in Eva Selhub's and Alan Logan's wise and penetrating *Your Brain on Nature*, "forest bathing" can reduce the stress hormone, cortisol, and increase the immune defence system. I loved the image of spreading out my arms and inhaling the scents of tall trees, of basking in their leafy splendor on a sunny day. A walk in the park could mean increased cerebral blood flow and improved mental health. The perfect antidote for someone recovering from a brain attack.

Robert Louis Stevenson wrote: "It is not so much for its beauty that the forest makes a claim upon men's hearts, as for that subtle something, that quality of air, that emanation from old trees, that so wonderfully changes and renews a weary spirit."

Even now, two years on, I still walk daily amongst trees to feel their healing powers. Nobody knows for sure the full extent of those powers, only that a daily walk in the companionship of trees is a gift that replenishes us.

Although the weekly routine of out-patient therapy was monotonous, the benefits I experienced over the next eight weeks were immeasurable. Each day contained a small but significant surprise. My foot suddenly bent at the ankle and I was able to lift my toes, ever so slightly, as if like plant shoots they'd felt the warmth of sunlight. Or I was finally able to pronounce a word without confusing the order of the vowels and consonants. Or I would look in a mirror and see my mouth form a straight line rather than a jagged downward slash across my face that made me look as though I'd lost a sword duel.

My therapists taught; I relearned.

I went from struggling in a wheelchair to walking, somewhat unsteadily, but walking all the same, with the aid of a walker and then a cane. At least for a few steps. What an accomplishment! Only in retrospect did I realize how repetitive and yet fruitful the various stages of recovery were.

Occasionally there were relapses. Even though I had passed the swallow test, I sometimes forgot to concentrate on what I was doing. When I went to the cafeteria with Pat or with a visitor for lunch, if I didn't focus on chewing and swallowing, if I got distracted by the conversation or if a comment upset me, food and drink went down the wrong pipe. Then I would aspirate, which would end in a violent fit of coughing. It was difficult to admit to anyone that I was still relearning something that had been habitual to me for as long as I had memory. The thought of returning to another form of feeding terrified me.

If I talked too much and for too long, I grew weary; and with fatigue, my speech became mangled, as if my tongue were being fed through a meat grinder.

My emotional control was fragile. When I viewed scenes of African, Asian or Latin American poverty, voiceless kids searching through the garbage of those in power or walking along streets flowing with sewage, I was angered and hurt. I would begin to weep at the most carefully staged funding ads of children in distress. Advertisements asking for donations were the worst. Even today, almost two years after my stroke, the slightest injustices provoke tears. My throat tightens, my speech becomes strained and I worry that someone may catch me on the verge of screaming out my anger. Restraint has become difficult. But more to the point, *why* do I worry about how others react to me and to what I think? Someone has to find the words to embody the dreams and nightmares of the world's homeless. They are so timid, so fearful, so silent.

And so alone.

Manic moments were just as common. The silliest jokes or slapstick incidents could send me into a torrent of unstoppable giggles. I felt transparent, almost indelicate. But not quite.

My therapy team — I say "my" because I think each one of the rehab patients claimed them as their own — was a dream. Deb pushed me to recover muscle strength. There was nothing unique about her exercise regimen — I pedalled a stationary bike, did leg lifts, climbed steps, stood on one leg then the other, did squats, arm pulls — exercises for both my paralyzed leg and arm, always with the wheelchair at hand or a safety harness around my waist. It was her encouragement and gentle method of persuasion, though, which worked wonders. On her instruction and with considerable effort, I happily took to a prone position on the floor, but once there, beached like a small sea lion, I wondered how in the name of all things holy I was going to get back to my feet. I envisioned them having to bring in a hoyer, the medical version of a hoist, to raise me back to my feet. Then she showed me how to roll over, a simple task before my stroke, and use the muscles on my good side to manoeuvre onto my knees and scramble onto one of the many therapy benches scattered around the gym. Each time I felt breathless from exertion and fear. You might think exertion was what I would remember most, the clambering, the scuttling like a crab, but what stuck most in my mind was fear. The sheer terror of being "disabled." Something Bonnie Sherr Klein describes with such clarity and poignancy in her *Out of the Blue: One Woman's Story of Stroke, Love and Survival.*

With each passing day I relearned movements that were as common as love and pain but sometimes as easily misunderstood.

Barb spent much of her time working on my swollen hand. It had puffed up to double its normal size. Like a blowfish. Blood and fluids were not flowing properly through my system; my lymph nodes were not working. When I accidentally fell, touring our garden, my first major outing with only my cane and Pat's assistance, and tried to break the fall with my right hand, I was certain I had broken my wrist. I remember sitting amongst the lavender and ornamental grasses, bellowing like a castrated bull.

X-rays and CAT scans of my wrist revealed nothing out of the ordinary, but the swelling persisted. And the pain, the mind-numbing pain, became the one constant in my new life. My fingers were fixed in a claw. Barb tried to encourage movement with electrical stimulation by attaching electrodes to related muscles and giving me a jolt, but with little success. Eventually the physiatrist gave me cortisone and Botox shots, one to lessen the pain, the other to loosen my shoulder. The pain eased and eventually my arm showed slightly more flexibility.

Minor victories.

Occupational therapy was a mix of exercises from threading nuts off and on bolts, to turning a steering wheel pilfered from a bus, to pushing and pulling a large and heavy wooden sledge, to trying to remove and replace small objects from a box, to playing electronic games. Wii, the name of the game or platform, I think, included bowling and soccer played on a TV screen with an imaginary opponent. I kicked at and threw an invisible ball, and the computer eye decided how accurate I had been. On reflection, I think electronic games could have been one of the more beneficial rehab tools, for three reasons: they tested my balance, our sixth sense and crucial to my making my way back into the world; they challenged my brain and physical recovery and development simultaneously; and they were fun. The random "cheery" and carefree minute or two of relief from the tedium of being captive to all the side effects of paralysis did wonders for my spirits. Increasingly, in my view, it was the symbiotic relationship of mind and body that was most significant in all forms of therapy.

Barb also had me refinish a wooden stool, first by sanding it down to bare wood and then by applying several coats of varnish. I was proud of this project but disappointed that I ended up doing most of the work with my left hand. My right hand simply couldn't hold the sandpaper or brush.

Slowly, oh so slowly, my arm regained some limited movement, yet I don't think Barb was ever satisfied with my progress. Or lack thereof. When she attempted to slide my hand up a door jamb to a position above my head the pain was excruciating, and I yelped and moaned. On one occasion I thought I was going to black out. At the time, I felt as though my failure to perform this "next step" indicated that I wasn't putting in enough effort. I feared censure. While I liked Barb, she was a kind and compassionate person, she could also be stern and uncompromising. Maybe she figured pushing limits was a necessary evil if I was to recover, but later, when I had a CAT scan done on my shoulder, we saw that everything was mangled: muscles, ligaments, cartilage and bone. A messy mass of bone and tissue perhaps left over from my rugby days. The physiatrist suggested I might have a frozen shoulder, not uncommon after a stroke.

Why, oh why, I wondered, did they not communicate more with each other?

As promised, after I'd been an out-patient for a few weeks, a district nurse came to do an evaluation of our house — was it suitable for someone who was handicapped — and to assess whether or not we were coping with my "altered circumstances." The euphemisms built around all forms of physical loss never cease to amaze me. My brother Brian, who wears a patch over the eye that was removed during his cancer operation, constantly fields pirate comments. A waitress, trying to be clever, once asked him in mid-July if he wasn't rushing Halloween. You never become accustomed to such thoughtlessness, he told me; you mend quickly and carry on. As if brushed by the shadow of a crow.

The district nurse arrived on the same day as Pat and I were discussing whether or not to renew the rental of the wheelchair. I think there were two or three days left on the old agreement before we would have to sign a new monthly contract. By now I was getting around fairly well with a walker, and Pat felt the wheelchair was somewhat redundant. I still used it to sit in at the dining-room table or in front of the TV, but it was more a convenience than a necessity. I think by this time I viewed it mostly as an extension of my condition; it had become a prop, an addiction of sorts, one I needed to be rid of. Pat was concerned about the cost, one of many that had been added to our normal expenses. The medications took the heaviest financial toll. We are still debating in this country whether or not pharmaceuticals should be covered under universal health care.

But she was right. I no longer needed the wheelchair. Since late January, early February, we had been taking daily walks through the neighbourhood. I toddled along using the walker, Pat pushed the empty wheelchair. Just in case. Dressed in my black, heavy-woolen coat, I felt warm and resolute on those nippy, late-winter walks. I had decided to match Pat's steadfastness and not resort to the chair. I was determined to impress upon myself, her and our neighbours, who I figured must be watching me from behind their closed blinds, that I was a fighter. I would walk again unassisted and for long distances. But from the beginning and in spite of my defensiveness, paranoia and irrational posturing, my neighbours were never anything but kind and supportive. When we met in the street they greeted me with deference and always remarked on how well I was doing. They were quick to point out that they could see that I had made significant progress. I was pretty sure they weren't just saying this out of pity, which never helps. Their eyes, which I looked into as if into a wishing well, were sincere.

Just before the doorbell rang, Pat and I made up our minds. We decided to forgo the wheelchair. Pat, in particular, was pleased with this decision. We would be rid of a major reminder of what the stroke had done to me. Returning it was a powerful symbol of my recovery, one that gave our spirits, together, an enormous lift, as if we had found an affirmation that might just cheat what initially I had thought of as my fate.

As soon as the district nurse passed through the door and settled into a chair in the living room, I sensed that we were not going to get along. I'm not sure what got my hackles up, but right away I distrusted her and was on the defensive. For no apparent reason. Although in retrospect there was something about the way she moved that troubled me. When she removed her shoulder bag and started to rummage inside it, every movement, accompanied by a weary sigh, was laboured, as if what she carried in the bag was leaden; as if she was burdened by all the serious and weighty troubles of the world. She was one of those people of an indeterminate age, somewhere between thirty and fifty, who projected a gloomy self-assurance. Right away I felt I wouldn't know whether to take her advice seriously or nod my head and wait for another opinion.

I was astonished by my prejudice. Why was I reacting to her this way? Since the stroke, Pat had noticed that with time I was becoming much more tolerant and unflappable. Or at least that was what we both thought. My old restless self, sometimes volatile or cynical, had either departed or was hidden in a remote and perhaps damaged part of my brain.

Pale winter sunlight shone through the French doors and glistened on a patch of the nurse's mousey-brown hair like a light dusting of snow. Dust motes danced above her head. She reminded me of a prim TV mother, the sort of officious character I had watched and rebelled against all my life.

She asked me to recount my stroke story. How had it happened? Where was I when it happened? What did I feel when it happened? How did I feel *now* about what had happened to me? Did I feel resentment? Depressed? How was my therapy going? All questions I had answered countless times before and didn't want to answer yet again. Certainly not to another stranger.

Then she took an inventory of all the medical aids we had borrowed from the Red Cross. She asked if we were aware of the various stroke groups in the area. When we both shook our heads, she was shocked and suggested we might want to check them out. We might find them useful. Associating with other stroke survivors might be beneficial, might be a source of useful advice about coping with my new body and the new me. As far as she was concerned, the lessons and experiences of other stroke victims were the most valuable resource available. And right at my fingertips. Free.

While I didn't doubt this was the case, I told her, I was ready and hoping, at least for the time being, to spend some of my spare time on my own. Either resting or doing additional therapy. When I told her I received my fill of "stroke rehab advice" every day during therapy at the hospital, she looked at me over the top of her glasses as if I were one of the most insensitive and ungrateful lunkheads she'd ever met.

As she continued her well-rehearsed talk, she rocked to and fro and hugged her knees as if the rhythm of this motion brought her comfort and confidence.

Then she suddenly stood, as if shot out of a whale's blowhole or, perhaps more accurately, had been released from some sort of grievous bondage, and asked if we would mind giving her a tour of the house. In particular she wanted to see the "bathing arrangements."

There we go again, I thought: "bathing arrangements!" The language was taking a battering.

She seemed pleased with what she saw.

"The shower is very accessible, although you," she said turning to me, "might have difficulty climbing in and out of the bathtub." Then turning to Pat and clearly assuming I was both bumbling and too simple to understand what she was about to say, she said, "Do you know that you're eligible for housekeeping assistance? Up to a point. There are limits, of course. As with most government programs."

"No 'we' didn't," I made a point of answering.

"Do you use the commode in the shower?"

She now glared at me.

"I used to, but I'm trying to make do with the indoor walker," I said proudly. "I stand when I shower. In the long term, I'm hoping to walk without any aids."

But instead of giving me encouragement, as all the other therapists made a point of doing, she examined me as if I were a misguided optimist. A deluded fool.

I hated her look of self-importance and self-belief.

Then she asked me about the wheelchair, which I had noticed her eyeing since her arrival.

"Are you planning to keep the chair?"

"No," I said emphatically, "no, I don't think so. It's time to wean myself off of it as well."

"In fact," Pat injected, "earlier today we decided to return it. As a token of Ron's recovery."

"Oh," the district nurse said with a note of regret, "oh, I wouldn't be quite so hasty. You never know."

She looked at me as if she were looking at a child who needed scolding.

"By now you may have recovered as much as you're going to. Strokes are very difficult. And unpredictable."

I was flabbergasted. Who had endured the stroke here? What could she possibly know about living inside a stroke?

"You mustn't be in a rush to get rid of your wheelchair," she continued, "recovery is rare." And here she paused as if what she had to say next she wanted to make even more theatrical.

"You might well be in it for the rest of your life!"

Much to my surprise, she said this with an air of anticipatory triumph.

"You might want to reconsider your decision. At least until you know your circumstances for certain."

That was it! At no other point in my life had I felt so betrayed.

As far as I was concerned, she was flat-out wrong. I wanted nothing to do with "naysayers." I wanted to say to her, "Get out of my house!" but I didn't. Instead I refused to answer any more of her insipid questions. I took heart from Sarah's mother in *Left Neglected* when she told Sarah, "nothing's impossible."

Soon the district nurse took the hint, handed us a few pamphlets from her bag and prepared to leave.

I was furious and saddened. I had just had my first encounter with someone who seemed to derive perverse pleasure from casting me in the role of "the handicapped." And herself, perhaps (am I being unkind?), as the Queen of Sheba.

In mid-March my placement in intensive out-patient therapy came to what I considered an abrupt end. To be fair, this end was not unexpected. I had been forewarned. At the very beginning of therapy, at one of the meetings where we had discussed the particulars of my rehab program, I had been told by "the team" the exact date when my time as an out-patient would be terminated. I was flummoxed. How on earth could they anticipate, let alone calculate, my progress with such precision? In fact, I had managed to wheedle two additional weeks from Elvira by claiming I was being short-changed because of the extra time staff were taking off for their Christmas holidays.

My tactics were shameless, trying to play on her guilt to eke out a few more hours of treatment; playing the broken-body-and-mind card. As my roommate had done on the fourth floor, I was learning how to get my own way.

Even so, when the day came for my release, prematurely as far as I was concerned, I felt conflicted. I was both contrite and resentful, an odd emotional conundrum. Once again I was confused. I bounced back and forth between gratitude and anger. Mixed with a generous measure of hopelessness. Perhaps depression. I could no longer distinguish between the two. Everyone kept suggesting greater independence was good for my morale.

In whose opinion, I wondered?

I thought differently.

Wouldn't a period of transition make more sense?

I considered my release a sign of indifference and carelessness.

Wasn't the goal here to maximize recovery?

I wanted continued attention from those whose expertise would help me to regain mobility, from those who presumably understood the mechanics and treatment of muscles, bones and the nervous system in recovery.

I realize, of course, that when I say "abrupt" I mean that *I* wasn't ready to leave the program. I didn't feel my rehabilitation was complete. Far from it. I felt as though I was on the verge of making significant progress in returning to normal. I had all sorts of grandiose plans. Any day now I expected to leap to my feet, do a cartwheel, followed by a couple of handsprings, and sprint off into the distance. I would become a mere speck on the horizon where I would resume my life as an able-bodied member of the human race. I would become a bona fide hominoid once again.

And yet . . .

More and more I doubted my resilience.

Who was I kidding?

Perhaps everyone who suffers brain trauma and paralysis feels there is more healing to be accomplished, that the sudden termination of therapy sends a message of premature finality.

You have reached a dead end, a cul-de-sac, the brink, the cliff's edge of recuperation.

Allowable or prescribed therapy appeared to have a strict timetable, one that seemed totally arbitrary and out of sync with patients' actual recovery, one, I suspect, that had been dreamt up in some remote corner of an administrative tower. Shades of Kafka. This quota said, "We can no longer justify your therapy as a productive use of our time and resources." Suddenly it occurred to me that I was being "turned out" as a cost-saving measure.

These days even miracles had become a subject for cost-benefit studies.

This was maddening. I *was* making progress. Four months after my stroke, I was getting about solely with the aid of a walker. Not for great distances, mind you, half a mile at best, and then I felt exhausted and ready for a nap, but I had graduated from lying paralyzed in bed to threading my way ever so slowly for a few hundred feet up our gravel driveway, around potholes, over curbs and down the paved road that circled past our house.

I was no longer shackled to memories or imaginary feats of derring-do such as sailing around the world on a raft *à la* Pi or crossing the Salish Sea in a hot-air balloon; I was a free spirit again, ready to shuffle slowly and abidingly through a world of endless wonders and challenges.

But I was being "terminated."

To be on my own; I was now frightened in a brand new way.
How was I going to cope?

I don't think anyone but other stroke survivors understands or appreciates the fear you feel after your brain has been bombed and you have struggled to regain a semblance of normality with only moderate success. You are frozen in time and space, your gaze focused on a multitude of possibilities, wondering in which direction salvation lies. Fear is your guide, solidarity with the rest of the world your goal, that goal a small receding dot in the distance.

Perhaps we need to concentrate more on what it means to be healthy.

Perhaps we need to concentrate more on wellness than illness.

Perhaps we need to recognize that the word "remembered" is as important as the word "forgotten."

Many months later, long after I had left the hospital, I had a chance to reflect on my therapy experience. First of all, what a difficult job therapists have, especially on a stroke ward, caring for a motley band of "over-the-hill," "down-in-the-mouth" wrecks trudging from one calamity to the next.

That said, I think the treatment protocols were far too prescriptive. Most of the therapists appeared to consult the same training manual. In my case, no one ever asked me what was going on inside my mind. My brain.

I admit, I'm not quite sure how you search the byways of the brain, but someone needed to do it, perhaps a neuropsychologist. As far as I'm concerned, ignoring the brain and the patient's personal "story" was a critical oversight. Stroke attacks the whole person, the spirit as well as the body.

To be fair, my therapists did ask me how I was doing, in the same way they might ask the victim of a highway or sporting or domestic accident or a hip or knee replacement patient how they were getting on. There was never a shortage of compassion. But an assault to the brain is supposed to be unique to each patient and should not be treated as commonplace. The answers to vital questions will never be the same and therefore need individual interpretation.

All forms of stroke therapy should evaluate a patient's strengths as well as her or his weaknesses. To a certain extent, in my case, that was done. But the therapy I received addressed only the physical side of my rehabilitation. The evaluation ended with: "Oh, he's paralyzed. Let's get him on his feet." Instead, I think the therapists needed to identify everything that was still working, physically and mentally. They had to find at the outset of therapy what was still there in me, what was my personal narrative, what could be developed, what could be encouraged, what could lead to an understanding of my specific needs. Affirming strengths feeds the desire as well as the ability to heal.

No exercise, whether physical or cognitive, will benefit the patient if not built on the patient's strengths. I felt the therapy I received dealt with only half of the problem. Those working on my recovery needed to see the healthy side of me, nurture and protect that, while treating what was broken.

Don't get me wrong, I'm indebted to my therapists, they got me up and walking and that was a huge achievement. But I wonder what they could have accomplished if they had known what was going on inside my head.

Therapy should build on strength, not just dwell on loss.

Recently I was rereading John Berger's short essay "Ape Theatre" in his 1991 collection, *Keeping a Rendezvous*. In this short piece he gives what could be a description of the dilemma stroke survivors face when they receive "physical-only" therapy. He writes: "Mostly, the thinkers of the nineteenth century thought mechanically, for theirs was the century of machines. They thought in terms of chains, branches, lines, comparative anatomies, clockworks, grids. They knew about power, resistance, speed, competition. Consequently, they discovered a great deal about the material world, about tools and production. What they knew less about is what we still don't know much about: the way brains work. I can't get this out of my mind: it's somewhere at the centre of the theatre we're watching." (145)

"The way brains work," he writes. This is the key to the theatre Berger is witnessing.

For the past two hundred years we've looked at the body as a machine, from the mechanical and scientific side of things, all in the service of the industrial and capitalist revolutions. The corporate and military complexes. As we take the next technological leap, specifically in electronics, digitization and artificial intelligence, what we have proclaimed as progress, perhaps we need to stop and reconsider. Perhaps now is when we need to rediscover what we once knew intuitively about our innate consciousness, the source of metaphor and of our knowing our place in the cosmos. That, I believe, will start us on the path to knowing "the way brains work," which in my view lies somewhere at the centre of stroke rehabilitation.

TEN

Fragments: Searching for Normality

In 2002, Dr. Douglas F. Watt of the Quincy Medical Center, Boston School of Medicine, wrote: "One might add parenthetically that despite all the advances in neuroscience, our hands-on clinical management of the regrettably commonplace problem of strokes has not advanced much at all in the past 200 years." (392) Robert McCrum came to a similar conclusion in his 1998 book, *My Year Off: Rediscovering Life after a Stroke*: "Doctors hate an illness they cannot cure, which is part of the explanation for the profound and chronic neglect of stroke-patients. (In many provincial hospitals, the out-of-the-way bed at the end of the ward is often still referred to as the 'stroke bed'.)" (117) On reflection, I thought I had occupied that bed on the fourth floor of the Nanaimo Regional General Hospital in the room I shared with my irksome roommate, the one whose wild conspiracy theories made anything seem possible. Even normal.

Over a dozen years later, I worried there was still a disquieting measure of truth to the observations made by Watt and McCrum. Despite major discoveries and exciting predictions about the "workings" of the brain through recent research into brain plasticity and hugely successful advances in endovascular therapy used in stroke treatment, I was convinced not much of that knowledge had seeped down to stroke wards, especially in the typical regional or rural hospital.

To compound the problem, little is known about the finer complexities of the brain. Yes, we understand the motor locations within the brain, we know where the speech centres are, and we know what each hemisphere does. We understand which cognitive test is most appropriate for certain types of strokes. And CT or MR images show very precisely where the damage has occurred in the brain from the stroke or infarct. And yet we know little about thoughts, memories, dreams and so on, all the remarkable functions of the brain. We really do not know how those might have been affected by a stroke.

As I read these and other stroke accounts after my release from rehab, I wondered: What's to be done? I felt abandoned, not by my family and friends who continued to encourage me in every possible way, but by a system that appeared to have contrived an arbitrary treatment program, one that conformed to the rules of ledgers — debits and credits — and not to medical protocols and potentially life-changing research. Those on the team were cutting me off, pleasantly enough, but aborting me all the same. Smile, I thought.

And at a time in my recovery when I didn't quite yet know where or who I was. Certainly not in any complete sense. Smile again.

Caught in a strange sort of limbo, not knowing if I had achieved what "the team" expected from me or if I was an inept, cack-handed failure, incapable of further rehabilitation, I felt betwixt and between. Was I simply to continue doing the exercises I had been stumbling through for the previous four months? Or was I to search out alternative forms and places of therapy? No one seemed to have a plan. When I asked, I was greeted with a lot of shoulder shrugs and hemming and hawing. Everyone grew mute, not with indifference, but yearning. Most health professionals take an oath to which they feel loyal. And I was convinced that my therapists felt uncomfortable with my leaving the program. I think to a person they thought they could advance my recovery, perhaps not have me running marathons, but at least have me ambling freely up a mountainside or along a forest path or over a rocky shoreline.

I needed time. Termination of therapy seemed totally arbitrary.

Now, as it happened, I still relied on my walker, but I could get about the house with my cane. My leg and arm still suddenly and unexpectedly shuddered with spasms, sometimes violently, always painfully.

When I complained of extreme pain and increasing tightness in my right shoulder, the physiatrist gave me a second cortisone shot and suggested another Botox injection. At close to a thousand dollars a shot, I wasn't keen and said no. I hadn't noticed significant improvement after the first pokes with a rather long needle.

My family doctor, Dr. Steyn, who told me he had come to the hospital on a couple of occasions only to discover me sleeping soundly and therefore had let me be, took over my care and quickly adjusted my medications. I think he wanted to reassure me that he had been attentive to my condition; and I think he was concerned about the number of drugs I was taking and the dosages. (He's a knowledgeable and caring man, who is both unsentimental and quick to admonish me when I don't heed his advice. Now I wished I had listened to him earlier. Perhaps this stroke experience could have been avoided. Hindsight is nothing but wishful thinking delayed.) I was pretty certain statins were causing me all sorts of grief and he suggested going off them for a while.

"But," he added, "I think you've been receiving excellent care."

I agreed.

And yet . . . and yet, I was being set adrift like an origami boat placed in a stream to see which way the currents flowed.

I was being asked to find my own way, which was a little like confiscating a blind man's cane and setting him down in the middle of a maze.

This sudden and forced independence was an intimidating proposition. Alone I had to dare to see what worked. To see what could be recovered.

I still knew little about how to rehab my own body. I knew what needed work — virtually every muscle on my entire right side had lost mass, movement and strength. My shrivelled right leg and arm still hung like bent limbs on a scarecrow — a light breeze would have knocked me over — and my midriff had pooched. I felt like I lived in a world where "I," the old "me," was at risk of being lost. What was visible and remembered existed, what was unseen and forgotten didn't. Perhaps this process of acknowledging and ignoring had always been in play, had always been the case, but now I seemed to belong to a "way of being" that was in a constant state of reduction. My world was getting smaller and me with it.

In the first few weeks on my own, I continued doing variations on the exercises I had been doing at the rehab centre. Simple bends and squats, exercises to fight flexion (the tendency of muscles to curl up and resist extension), especially in my arm and fingers. Occasionally I ventured up and down the stairs between the two levels of our house, each trek ending with me clutching the railing, and gasping and straining to reach the top landing. Climbing took every ounce of energy I could muster. Sixteen stairs in total, stairs I had been able to skip up and down two at a time before my stroke.

I took daily walks with Pat, shambling along behind my walker as if I were pushing a pram that required my full concentration and attention, down Evanshire, our neighbourhood street, each day adding a few feet to the distance we travelled, each day chalking up a little victory on the road to recovery. After weeks of being cloistered in the rehab unit, I relished every breath of cool spring air, greedily gulping in the fresh, moist scents of budding plants and freshly turned mulch, perhaps another form of forest bathing.

Then two things happened, both of which gave my recovery much needed direction and impetus.

As the pain in my shoulder persisted (the cortisone had helped a bit) and my wrist, hand and fingers had ballooned like ripening melons, Marg James, Gerry's wife, wondered aloud one day over a cup of coffee if I might not benefit from a few sessions of acupuncture.

"You never know, it might help. It's definitely helped me with the neuropathy in my feet and legs. And the woman I go to, Elaine, is a real character and very good. You'll like her, in spite of the needles, which I have to confess no longer bother me."

Marg was right, Elaine was a special breed. At seventy-nine, she had the energy of a woman half her age and the inquisitiveness of a young girl. She looked at you as if she were examining you on a slide under a microscope, although she was too artful and far too busy to make this embarrassing. Behind her thick glasses, her eyes roamed, forever seeking interesting places to land.

And land she would, needle at the ready.

She loved to talk, her voice flitting about like a butterfly from one subject to another, from places she had been, to the genius behind a musical score she was studying, to the discipline and precision it took to insert each needle at the precise point on the right meridian — channels of energy running the length of the body — to find and achieve a balanced *qi*. "How you rotate and direct the needle is important," she said. Her words soothing, reassuring.

I listened for a promise of less pain.

For years Elaine had suffered chronic migraines, throbbing pain that was so severe she eventually had to quit her job as a high-school science teacher. Leaving the classroom was difficult. For a woman who had studied in Paris and taught in Germany, sharing knowledge was a passion.

Traditional Western medications provided no relief from her

persistent headaches. On the advice of a friend (and as a last resort), she went for acupuncture treatments. At that stage she had nothing more to lose.

To her surprise and delight, the acupuncture treatments worked! For the first time in years she was free of pain. In fact, she was so impressed with the results, she packed her bags and journeyed to China where she studied and voluntarily practised the art of acupuncture for two years under a well-known master in Beijing.

Perhaps I'm exaggerating her story here, but this is what I recall her telling me as I sprawled out on the table like a porcupine.

Sometimes my brain still plays tricks on me.

Filled with anticipation and enthusiasm, Elaine returned to Nanaimo where she set up her own small practice down by the waterfront, in a small windowless space divided into three rooms. Her office was messy but functional, an evolving project. Inside these walls, she told me, she dreamt of helping people, of relieving them of pain.

One day Pat and I arrived to find her standing over a large open cardboard box of plastic bones and illustrated instructions she had tossed on the floor.

"I don't need those. I know where everything goes," she said.

This full-sized human skeleton complemented the various charts she had pinned to the wall, each providing a different map of the human body. The most important chart showed the forty-one cardinal points used in acupuncture.

Her treatment table, set up in a small separate room, was like countless other therapy tables I'd seen, too high off the ground for someone with a handicap to reach. With an assortment of books, Elaine improvised a stair and, with her help, I managed to climb on top and stretch out on a linen sheet pulled over a vinyl mattress. As she chatted away she inserted needles in my feet, knees, wrists, arms and shoulders, a couple to relax me, several others to treat the tightness and pain in my right leg, arm and shoulder.

On subsequent visits, she attempted to treat the severe edema, or swelling, in my wrist and hand.

I have no idea how often I went for treatments, but in time the pain in my shoulder subsided and the swelling in my wrist lessened. What I remember best about Elaine was how concerned she was for me and how keen she was to treat me. She even opened her office on Good Friday so that I wouldn't go too long between sessions. Any measure of improvement in my condition pleased her, as if she had solved once again a mystery about how energy flows through the body.

So, while the acupuncture was helping my shoulder and hand, the second thing that changed after I had been banished from organized therapy, and that made a huge difference to my sense of recovery, was reading. At long last, I could prop a book up on my clenched right fist and turn pages with my left hand. Reading — what a luxury, a joy, a reaffirmation — what a feast for a reawakening mind!

Before I had my stroke, my world had been one of books, gardening, travel and golf (which Mark Twain is supposed to have described as "a good walk spoiled"). I considered myself a fortunate man. Books, in particular, had been central to my life, as an English teacher, publisher, editor and scribbler. I would have liked to have been adept at drawing, but I always got sidetracked attempting to replicate precisely what I was looking at. I didn't want to stray from the original. Lines would get tighter and deeper and the drawing smaller, winding in on itself. It seemed the visual took place in the verbal part of my brain and wouldn't allow my wrist and fingers to hold a pencil loosely to flow over paper free of inhibition. Prior to my stroke, I had often wondered if my neural pathways were crossed at birth. After my stroke, I wondered if some reconfiguration might take place. It didn't, I still translated what I saw into words.

As a reader you develop empathy for the work of certain writers. When I was a student at Leeds, I felt a special kinship with Jonathan Swift and Samuel Beckett. Towards the end of my studies, when Pat and I were planning a train trip to the former Yugoslavia to visit old friends, one of my professors handed me an introductory letter to Beckett who, when I landed in Paris several weeks later on our return trip to London, I was supposed to phone and arrange to meet. This would have been in 1970. I left the letter in my suitcase. I was terrified by the idea of speaking directly to the author who in one of his plays had a character say "Crrrritic" with such contempt. And who was the creator of Murphy, Malone and Malloy — amazing and somewhat crackpot representatives of humanity.

My lack of self confidence got in the way of what could have been a memorable day. A few years later I learned from a colleague who was given a similar letter of introduction by the same professor that she had spent a wonderful day with Beckett, walking from one sidewalk café to another, drinking wine in the Paris sun. All I'm left with is a title for a short story, "The Day I Didn't Meet Samuel Beckett." What a shame. Not even a trace of the "moment that wasn't" remains, not even the letter of introduction.

"The number of lives that enter our own is incalculable."

In recent years I have devoured the works of John Berger, an author whose writing resonates with me on every level imaginable. Would I fear his formidable intelligence in the same way as I had Beckett's? I hope not, his voice is gentle, sensual, concerned. He tries to bring sense to a world that is terribly off kilter, which is a little wobbly on its moral axis.

While in hospital, a new writer entered my life. My mother, who knew I loved Italy, brought me a copy of *Every Day in Tuscany* by Frances Mayes. My mother's name is also Frances, which may have been the initial attraction.

"I liked as much of her as I was able to read," my mother told me, "but the print was too small and I gave up on the book. Why don't publishers use larger type, especially for us older folk?" she asked. "You should know the answer to that!"

As a publisher myself, I think she felt I should respond to her complaint on behalf of the entire print and publishing industries.

As it turned out, *Every Day in Tuscany* was the first book I was able to hold and read after my stroke. Why didn't publishers make books lighter and easier to hold with just one hand? And while they were at it, they could invent a way to hold the book and flip pages with the same hand! (No, to those who are likely to suggest it: ebooks were not a solution.)

Frances hooked me in a couple of pages. There was much to admire in her writing not least of which was her ability to transport me beyond the fetters of my handicap to inside the walled cities of Siena and Urbino and to the Po River flatlands of Ferrara, the city of bicycles.

I sent her a note through her blog:

> During my first weeks in hospital I was wondering what to do with my days, apart from work, towards a full recovery. At first, reading was out of the question; I simply could not hold a book. A few weeks into my rehab my mother came for a visit, she is 87 (her name happens to be Frances), and left behind a copy of *Every Day in Tuscany*. She knows my passion for Italy. So as soon as I could hold the book I began my journey. What a wonderful adventure it has been. Your writing is delicious: all the tastes, smells, sights, sounds, textures of rural and urban Italy are so vivid. I love your mix of memoir, recipes, travel, art history, landscape; I love the freedom of the writing, the layers, the music and dance of the language. I love the scatter so beautifully recalled. I was particularly pleased to hear your response to Ferrara, a town where friends of ours own a trattoria. Ironically his name happens to be Francesco.

I was also surprised to read C.D. Wright's name, a poet I much admire. When I was Fulbright Chair in Creative Writing at ASU I met her husband, Forrest Gander, another fine writer. Your book is full of so many wonderful surprises, so many tastes. Yes, a taste treat with just the right dash of wisdom, of thoughtfulness. Thank you for this gift. You have helped me immeasurably through a very difficult time. I was sad when the book finished; I was taking it in in such measured dollops. Ah, but you might say, I can go back, as I hope to do soon — to Italy.

I was delighted to receive this brief response Frances wrote to my posting:

Ron — It's wonderful that you have made such a recovery! Bravo!! Many thanks for all the kind words. Yes, C.D. Wright and Forrest Gander are such amazing writers. They are old friends from San Francisco. I hope to see you in the piazza one day very soon!!! Frances

This short exchange with Frances Mayes reconnected me to the world of books, a world that had played such a large role in my adult life. Reading for me offered an escape if not a reprieve from thinking about the flow of time, my weakness of body and my dying. I'd had enough of gloomy thoughts. As far as I was concerned, storytelling affirmed the cycle of life. Of "being." While there was no doubt life was short and was all too frequently filled with hardship and inexplicable cruelty, books for me championed the struggle to survive in the midst of opposing forces, a struggle often caused by selfishness, by displacement, by political stupidity or by corporate greed and power. They touched our boundless spirit and drive to seek the truth and spoke from the heart about our respect for the past and the dead. Books were about our love for the sanctity of life and the pain we often suffered in order to defend some matter of principle or honour in spite of the ubiquitous tyrannies or the personal rashness that confused the moment. Perhaps most important, books were about our hope for unborn generations to come.

Through Mayes I continued to reclaim and re-inhabit the person I had been. After my stroke, regaining what and who I loved was the therapy that reshaped and revivified me. (I hesitate to say "cured," because I'm not convinced that happens.) Reading, editing and eventually writing this book helped give me back my life; helped me regain, at least in part, who I had been before I had my stroke.

In *Here Is Where We Meet*, John Berger remembers one of his mentors who introduced him to books: "Neither of us, for different reasons, believed in literary explanations. I never once asked him about what I failed to understand. He never referred to what, given my age and experience, I might find difficult to grasp in these books . . . There was a tacit understanding between us that we learn — or try to learn — how to live partly from books. The learning begins with our looking at our first illustrated alphabet, and goes on until we die." (88)

From Berger I heard the reasons to read; from Frances I heard the call to attend to business in the piazza.

There is one thing I soon learned for certain: there is no time limit on stroke recovery. The old notion that there is a limited window of opportunity in which to achieve rehabilitation is simply false, whether it be three months, six months, one year, two years and so on. The rate of recovery for each individual, I suspect, will be as unique as the stroke they've suffered. After all, we are dealing with individuals here. When Jill Bolte Taylor says "expect full recovery," I agree with her, although there must be an allowance made for the individual nature of the stroke. Some strokes are more severe than others, and the time needed for the nervous system and brain to heal will take longer. Taylor tells us that it took her eight years to recover fully.

And I suspect it depends on how we define "full recovery." If we mean a total return to the person we used to be, identical in every respect, then I think it's likely we're in for a huge disappointment. I imagine "full" recovery in this sense rarely, if ever, happens. With the passing of time, even in the normal world, people change.

Robert McCrum takes a somewhat dimmer view of recovering the old self: "The conundrum of stroke recovery is that while one's conscious efforts are devoted to recovering one's lost self, the cruel fact is that this former self is irretrievably shattered into a thousand pieces, and try as one may to glue those bits together again, the reconstituted version of the old self will never be better than a cracked, imperfect assembly, a constant mockery of one's former, successful individuality." (151)

In contrast, Dr. J. Allan Hobson, professor emeritus of the Harvard Medical School, in an email I received on October 2, 2014, remarked: "I have lived with twelve years of handicap and have never been happier or more productive. You can quote me," he added.

I found his words inspiring and encouraging. He was saying: There is life after stroke, quality life, a comment that echoed my own view of recovery.

Dr. Hobson suffered a stroke to his brain stem, in some ways similar to mine, fourteen years earlier, while vacationing in the south of France. He was sixty-seven at the time. He then wrote a short and fascinating anecdotal account of his experience for the scientific journal *Consciousness and Cognition*. As a brain and sleep scientist, his subjective account echoed the sort of observations I had made, observations rarely recorded in "stroke talk." He was asking, amongst other things, for his colleagues to acknowledge the importance of non-empirical evidence in understanding the effects of stroke. It's worth quoting him at length, to underline the point I'm making about brain retraining as well as body retraining. Or therapy.

> To an outside observer, my recovery may appear complete. Some of my friends even prefer my now-leaner lines! But at 16 weeks poststroke, I am still aware of how far I have to go to

regain confident mobility, normal swallowing, and better control of salivation . . . I am nonetheless happy to be sleeping, dreaming, and engaging in other gratifying visceral behaviors even if all of these functions are distinctly altered — possibly permanently . . .

Subjective reports are always suspect but sleep science has learned to deal with them, in part, by correlating specific aspects of the reports with anatomical and physiological data. The common occurrence of strokes makes this approach both compelling and informative, especially if our misgivings about subjective data can be overcome. One way to do this is to record the subjective experience of stroke victims more aggressively, more thoroughly, and more systematically.

To accomplish this goal, neurologists need to be sensitized to the research significance and technique of subjective data collection. Family members are almost always available — and willing to help — as in my case. Hand-held tape recorders are inexpensive and can be used to augment dictated reports . . . (377–390)

Then Dr. Hobson explains why subjective accounts are so rare and sounds a cautionary note about saddling all stroke patients with the same diagnosis.

Several facts of modern medical life add to neurological short-sightedness in making such descriptions difficult to obtain. Because hospitals and doctors are so overburdened, hurried, and procedure-oriented and because hospital stays are so short, attention to psychological detail is likely to decline further rather than increase. And yet patients, like myself, have very little to do in hospitals except introspect! We thus need to take advantage of the availability of such privileged self-observation.

Otherwise in the absence of such affirmative action, the patient is reduced to a set of easily localized signs of CNS (central nervous system) damage and classic case status . . . (377–390)

Since we don't know exactly what a stroke is and tend to generalize, we can at least begin to record what it does to the individual patient's thoughts, emotions, and sense of self.

Some stroke survivors adapt, calling on an old skill to supplement or substitute for something they've lost after their brain has been bombed. Recently, I met a man named Joe in the hot tub at the local recreational facility where I go to exercise and to swim. After a few minutes of glancing back and forth across the bubbling froth, Joe asked me how I was doing.

"I've had a stroke," I told him.

"I know," he said, "I'm a retired physician."

"Two years ago," I added.

"You're doing well."

I was surprised by his matter-of-fact tone. Two years on, I liked to think the side effects, like getting warts from kissing a frog, were less obvious, especially while lounging in a hot tub, but he had probably noticed me floundering in the pool. And my cane leaning against a railing leading down the stairs into the hot tub was probably a dead giveaway — that and my drop foot, not to mention the flexion that returned to my right arm after a lengthy workout.

"The medical profession has never known much about strokes," he said, "but I still recognize the symptoms."

Then, after a few minutes of casual chatter, he said: "The way some people respond to their strokes has always struck me as rather remarkable. Human inventiveness is truly amazing."

Then he told me a story.

"Take, for example, the case of a patient of mine who woke up from his stroke totally paralyzed and unable to swallow or speak, yet in full possession of his cognitive powers, a not uncommon side effect of a brain attack, as you probably know. We — his family, friends, stroke specialists and nursing staff — we could all see in his eyes that he wanted to speak to us. And yet when he opened his mouth the best he could do was emit a sort of grunt. Then one day a family member noticed he was tapping a finger on his better side. He looked agitated and seemed to be annoyed with us. I'm not sure who saw it first, perhaps the speech therapist, but someone realized his tapping had a pattern to it. Then a family member blurted out that he had been a Morse code operator during World War II. He had found a way to speak to us. Eventually he made a full recovery, including his voice," Joe said, clearly pleased with this outcome, "although from then on he spoke less — as if he were saving something rare and precious."

Brain plasticity, I wondered. Does that include the ability to reduce what seems impossible to something a little less complicated?

My Irish friend, who suffered a fairly severe stroke ten years before I had mine, was determined to return to golf. He hired a personal trainer to help him with his physical recovery. Within two years he had gone from being paralyzed on his left side back to swinging a golf club. It helped that golf for him was a passion. He couldn't imagine living the rest of his life without the ritual of a round of golf at least three times a week. Twelve years later, at eighty-two, he was living his dream. But some things had changed. "I hit off the forward tees, which I used to think of as the "ladies tees," I slice the ball rather than hook it because of my weakened left side, and when I get home I need a nap. I'm still a little unsteady on my feet," he said, "but many Irishmen are." He winked and added, "I'm playing off a nine handicap, not bad for someone my age."

Modest changes, finite victories perhaps, but victories all the same.

What's particularly discouraging is the length of time recovery takes — discouraging for everybody, patients and therapists, not to mention the health system itself. We are a society that expects immediate results, and if those results are not achieved in a predictable time frame we scuttle the project or redefine the parameters of the process. We give up on the patient. Our model is the business model applied to a health issue. Cost benefit. We get caught up in statistics: the average time a survivor needs a bed; the likelihood of full recovery; the quick and slow of medical interventions and physical exercise; sleep time and the cost of staff. I'm not proposing that it's possible to recover from every stroke, some are simply too severe, but I saw too many examples of people who had been abandoned.

More effort and resources need to be expended on understanding the cognitive side of the damage done.

As I sit here at 6:00 a.m. jotting down these thoughts I'm reminded I'm only three months away from the second anniversary of my stroke. When I was released from rehab I was led to believe that I could still expect improvement in my condition but that the table had pretty much been set. Keep your expectations in check was implicit in what I was being told. Be reasonable. Don't hope for too much; you don't want to be disappointed. We know so little about strokes.

Why, I wonder? Why not imagine the improbable?

So, I ask again, what is a stroke?

Shortly after I was released as an out-patient, my next-door neighbour, Bernie Binns, returned home from his yearly winter sojourn in New Zealand. He is a retired physician, a specialist, a gynecologist-obstetrician. He spends just short of half of each year, from late October to early April, "down under" where his wife, Elaine (another Elaine), also a physician, prefers to live. She is an anaesthetist who took up a locum several years ago in the land of the Kiwi and the All Blacks, and fell in love with the country. She prizes her small garden there, in particular the many varieties of roses she can grow. And the village in which they live reminds her of the village she grew up in back in rural England. She likes the intimacy of the place: the specialty shops — butcher, baker, greengrocer, bookstore, pub — all within easy walking distance of their house, and the friendliness of the people. Now Elaine and Bernie shift back and forth between their two homes on islands in the two hemispheres.

Bernie, who has the distinction of being one of the few people born on the Falkland Islands, had heard about my stroke from mutual friends and came to see me as soon as he'd recovered from his jetlag. As we visited and talked, I realized he knew as little about strokes as any of the other medical people I'd talked to, a fact he readily acknowledged. Then he recounted his first lecture in neurology at Guy's teaching hospital, a part of King's College London School of Medicine, where he took his training. His professor had marched into the lecture theatre and delivered a short, compelling, but somewhat indirect and subjective overview of the mysterious workings of the brain.

"Good morning, ladies and gentlemen. I would like you to consider the following. This morning most of you crawled out of bed at the right time, put on your clothes in the right order, perhaps scrambled an egg and boiled water for tea, gathered your books, stepped out the door remembering to lock it behind you, and probably arrived at the hospital on foot, on a bike or by using some form of London transport. In doing so, you walked up the steps to the right station, put your hand into your pocket where you had several coins of different sizes and denominations. Without looking you were able to select the correct coins and put them into the vending machine to purchase the right ticket. The walking was done completely unconsciously, but you might have had to think briefly about the coins in your pocket. Then you made your way from the station to here. Have any of you asked yourselves how you managed this very complex series of events? In the next ten lectures I will try to give you some idea of how you accomplished them. Essentially performing these tasks without giving what you were doing a thought. I will warn you now that the subject is very complicated."

Then, somewhat dramatically, he had turned with a flourish and walked out.

I'm not sure what I expected from Bernie's recounting, but it reminded me once again that what we manage to do on a daily basis "without giving it a thought" is astronomical. The number of neurons involved in the coordination of every physical transaction is enormous, the stuff of science fiction.

How many calculations does it take to scratch an itch?

And in that inner space, I realized, we also have to cope with our emotions, desires, fears, anxieties, hopes, worries, passions, silences, losses, dreams, not to mention our unfurling thoughts always waiting just out of reach on the edge of some unknown dimension or universe.

Most of the time, I sensed, we are like sleepwalkers.

After Bernie's review of his first neurology class, I realized in simple survivor/layman terms what a stroke meant to me. Put simply, my brain in a curious way had been separated from my body. The "automatic" connection between the two had been severed. A relationship I had taken for granted all my life no longer worked. Suddenly I had to think my way through actions and calculations that hitherto I'd done by rote.

You are going to have to relearn much of what you once knew, I had repeatedly told myself. And relearning is not passive. Brain recovery, I had come to understand, is nothing like the healing of a flesh wound, where a scab forms, which in turn is eventually replaced by new skin. Recovery from a brain attack requires considerable effort, building and rebuilding, from plans far more intricate and labyrinthine than a detailed map of the heavens seen through the most powerful telescope.

For several months after I stopped acupuncture I went for massage therapy on a regular basis — about every two to three weeks. While the pain had lessened in my shoulder, the tightness in the joint had increased. I was slowly losing range of motion and I was afraid this loss might become permanent. My therapist, Lisa Watson, whose seven-year-old son, Jon-Robbie, was on the trail of Bigfoot, began our sessions by reviewing my stroke history. What sorts of things had I done in occupational and physiotherapy? Which exercises did

I think benefitted me? What medications was I on, and did I take any supplements? Lisa, who had a Bachelor's degree in biology and anatomy, felt our modern diet lacked certain essential vitamins and minerals. Soon she had me taking more pills, most of them intended to aid circulation by softening my arteries. With my permission, she often consulted her father, who was a medical practitioner in the Maritimes, about possible explanations and cures for my various complaints.

I enjoyed these sessions with Lisa, because I felt her deep massage of the fascia layer surrounding the muscles that collected in my shoulder cavity was actually working — and because I appreciated Jon-Robbie's quest. Each session included a summary of his most recent exploits and discoveries — his sighting of what looked like enormous footprints in the moss in the woods adjacent to his house or his unearthing of an old bone, perhaps discarded by Bigfoot after a feast (never mind the two large dogs the Watsons had) — and I loved his willingness to embrace a myth that the adult world had dismissed as silly and baseless lore.

I liked that he wanted to share his story with me and Pat — who had her own peculiar fascination with the apelike creature known in our area as Sasquatch. For thirty years she had been working on a novel in which Bigfoot and the "Chimp with the Human Brain" had paired up to confound science and the international media with their exploits in and around Wild Goose Bay. To support her belief she drew my attention to a recent newscast in which two women driving home at dusk after an evening at their local pub witnessed Bigfoot galumph across a major highway and disappear into the undergrowth.

To be honest, I still wanted to believe that anything was possible.

Lisa's massages were unlike anything I had imagined. With her strong fingers she dug deep into my flesh and muscle. This was not gentle manipulation. Nor was it soothing and blissful. Her treatments hurt, deep down, usually for a couple of days. As the pain subsided I noticed that my shoulder had just a bit more movement and my arm was a little less tight. Over time I began to remember the motion of my arm and shoulder from my past when I had played catch with Owen. The picture was still incomplete, but Lisa had jarred loose the memory of another possibility.

After each session stray strands of hair covered her forehead and her roundish cheeks were flushed with exertion. And she always wore a smile. She would have been upset if I hadn't seen some benefit from her work, if I hadn't returned her smile and thanked her for her gift.

Eight months after my stroke I had already learned that there was nothing smooth or predictable about stroke recovery. My mind was still capable of plumbing the deepest, darkest depths of despair. My mood swings could be exasperating. One minute I was the model of optimism: I took great joy in whistling to the robins and purple thrushes that populate our garden; the next minute I would be contemplating the end, whatever that might be. As the days and months ticked by, I feared that reeling in a likeness of my former self was akin to landing a forty-pound sockeye salmon that's determined to break free from a hook that's tied to the end of a twenty-pound test line. Unless you were very careful and played the line, the fish would cough up the hook and swim away.

Much to my amazement, Pat and I have become members of a local stroke recovery group. I'm not a joiner, but to my surprise I enjoy the company of other stroke survivors. I have to admit, at first I was puzzled by my attraction to them. In the past I would have felt awkward and terribly self-conscious in such company. Nervous and ill-at-ease. My tolerance for what I perceived as abnormal was shamefully unsympathetic. I was well blinkered, my gaze easily averted. But now, at times, I feel tears well up in my eyes when I look around the room because stroke survivors no longer know how, or feel a need, to hide anything. I know, they know, we all know what the others are going through. The emotional toll is massive and that's what none of us can control. We can help each other, everybody tries as best they can, but our ability to do so is limited.

The range of damage done is staggering. Three arrive in wheel-chairs and show few signs of awareness. Their eyes are dull, as if they've withdrawn to be in a safe place, and when we form a circle to perform our exercises they don't move. Balls and bean bags land at their feet. They don't move. Can't move. One drools; one strug-gles to watch our movements though his head swivels on his neck like a bobblehead doll; and the third inevitably falls asleep.

Others, just a few, walk in unaided and appear to be normal, whatever that is. They are the ones who can do most of the exer-cises the therapist leads us through.

I lie somewhere in the middle. Half of my body can do the arm and leg drills to music from the forties and fifties — Doris Day, Perry Como, Lawrence Welk — but the other half, the crippled half, lags behind, can perform only a small portion of most of the move-ments. My right hand won't reach beyond my shoulder, and when it attains that pathetic height, my arm aches and finally quits. There is no question; at these moments I feel dejected.

But I try; I gear up my mind to try. I visualize doing what I can't do. Watching the others has me convinced that one day I'll move as well as some of them.

The last time I attended a session with the group, Pat dropped me off early and I took a seat in the empty circle. Soon, one of the men who had always seemed upbeat came through the door, saw me, limped over and plunked himself down on the chair next to me. On a previous occasion he had told me a little about himself. He was younger than I was, he suffered his stroke a year before I experienced mine, he was married, and he had been a machinist all through his working life. He still had a shop in the village, filled with presses, punches, drills, lathes, milling machines, taps and dies, vises and clamps, acetylene torches, anvils and so on, thousands of dollars worth of equipment just lying there gathering dust, he said.

He obviously loved his shop.

We chatted and then out of the blue he whispered: "I wish I hadn't survived."

I was stunned. "You can't mean that," I said.

"I'm a burden. For my wife, for everyone I care about. I have a shop that no one wants. I'm obsolete. Everything is prefabricated these days."

"I'm sure that's not how your wife feels," I said. "Look at the recovery you've made. You're way ahead of me."

"Yes, but I can't run the machines. I don't have the strength. And my wife, she has to live with this. It's not fair to her."

I didn't know what else to say. The two of us sat there as the others trickled in. In a way he was asking me to answer a question for which I don't think there is an answer. The best I could do was listen. It's the unknown that's most threatening, even when the known seems unbearable.

In retrospect, I could have said more. But it occurred to me at the time how lucky I was. "My shop" was the world of books, and returning to the world of books had been relatively easy. To being a reader, editor and writer. And Pat shared my passion. I already knew how much therapy needed to include finding a way back to a semblance of the person you had once been. In my friend's case, the community had an invaluable source of information and skill. School kids could have benefitted from his knowledge and his shop. All it would have taken was the will and a little compassion. He would have loved to show kids his shop.

I'm not talking about just one person here; I'm talking about all stroke survivors who still have a role in society, a job they can do, a variation perhaps on the job they used to do. There is a need to find a place for them in their reconfigured worlds, a range of roles that will feed their need to feel both valuable and valued.

Listen, please, someone listen.

Now it is midsummer, nearing the end of July, and the arbutus are shedding their leaves. These are busy trees. Bernie tells me they shed something or other at least six times a year. Leaves, bark, berries, flowers, more leaves, and something of which I'm unaware. Stroke recovery is also busy. There is always something new happening. A twitch here, a twitch there, each bringing hope and more hope.

I tell myself I must keep this thought uppermost in my mind.

A few days ago, Pat and I joined a local recreational facility where I have access to a small weight room with dead weights, a stationary bike, a treadmill and various other instruments of torture I never use.

One day while walking on the treadmill a younger man working out across the room from me dropped his iPod on the frame of a stair stepper. When plastic hit metal my head whipped round and I almost blacked out. I staggered and hit the emergency stop button. The explosion continued to reverberate through the air as I grabbed on to Pat. My startle reflex caused me to turn so quickly my doctor is convinced I experienced whiplash. I have to get used to the fact that my hearing and sight are still extremely acute.

Sudden noises can be as dangerous as a concealed switchblade.

After working out for half an hour, travelling kilometres along poplar-lined lanes without leaving the premises and doing step-ups which would take me to at least the third floor of any respectable building without an elevator — did I mention that I plan to return to walk the cobbled streets of London, Rome and Paris — I reward myself with a swim in the twenty-metre pool.

Being in water is a special treat. Never before had I thought of swimming as defying gravity, but that is exactly what it is. Why hadn't I received water therapy before now? For the first time in ages I can lift my right arm without pain, I can run on the spot without fear of falling and I can float. What an incredible sensation

— floating, face down or on my back. Lately I have managed to swim, after a fashion, although Pat says I'm the only person she has ever seen do the crawl backwards. I tell her I don't really mind if I arrive feet first or hands first, as long as I have moved from one point to another. What's the old cliché? It's the journey that matters.

My right arm and hand, after several sessions, are actually breaking the surface of the water. I'm almost at the stage where enough of both rise above the water for me to turn my head and take a breath, a critical part of the mechanics of swimming. Breathing is a bonus, because it means laps are in my future. More importantly, I'm beginning to feel human. And a member of the aquatic fraternity.

Splashing about is quite primal. As I understand it, whales, dolphins, porpoises all have brains with brain-to-spinal-cord ratios larger than humans, which might, I've heard, say something about our respective intelligences. I feel very much as if I'm embracing something essential, a part of me I had forgotten, even before my stroke.

August 20, 2013. Nicole's birthday. Lately I have started to keep a diary of sorts. I see this as another way of reconnecting with my past. Today I read in the *New York Times* that Elmore Leonard, author of *Get Shorty* and *Hombre* amongst many other novels, had died from a stroke at the age of eighty-seven. I was saddened. He was a fine and gifted writer. He would have been critical of my abundant use of adverbs and shocked by my frequent use of "suddenly." But a stroke is like that; it is sudden and random, and shockingly debilitating. I've struggled to find a language that would tell my stroke story with the clarity and precision that characterized his prose style. Often I've had to skirt around my narrative, coming at it obliquely, through adverb, suddenly. Loss, pain, fatigue, change, doubts, unexpected shifts from ecstasy to despair define stroke. I hope he was spared these.

This morning as I climbed out of sleep, I found myself reflecting on the amount of sleep we "carbon units" need. The term comes from the 1960's TV show *Star Trek*, the brainchild of Gene Roddenberry, starring William Shatner as Captain James T. Kirk, Leonard Nimoy as Commander Spock, and DeForest Kelley as Dr. Leonard "Bones" McCoy. I liked the program and wished we had already advanced to that level in medicine where Bones would scan my head with some sort of sensor device (or was it his tricorder?), then run some other device over my damaged brain and I would be immediately healed.

I liked the program because of Roddenberry's utopian vision. In the 1960s and '70s, when the world was falling apart, again, he still held out hope. In his rendition of the future we were more interested in saving worlds than exploiting them or destroying them. We had no need for money. Race was no longer an issue, although some beings from our sector of space were still flexing muscles while others extolled our sense of tolerance and cooperation to those warring species from other universes, dimensions, sectors. Often these conflicts arose from complex misunderstandings. What's new? As much as Roddenberry thought outside the box, he was still in it. The ideals espoused in his interpretation of space were still grounded in his variant of an "ideal" America. In his version of the future we had reached our level of enlightenment only after escaping from the very precipice of annihilation. Even the stoical Spock (*Mr.* Spock?) emerged from an emotionally chaotic place, the planet Vulcan.

As the sun rose, my mind flitted and fluttered about like a moth to light, from one beautiful thought to another — from the real, to the impulsive, to the regretted, to the recalled, to the imagined.

Thinking has become a prized activity for me, probably because I realize how lucky I am that I can do it.

I sleep poorly. I rarely get through an entire night without some form of break. Consequently, during the day I fatigue more quickly than I used to. My failure to sleep is largely a consequence of the limited mobility of my right arm. And because my shoulder is still partially frozen, it is difficult to find a comfortable position in which to rest. Sometimes the pain is quite severe.

Oh for Bones's little whirling healer!

As much as I'd hoped to do so, I have come to realize that it's impossible to keep a complete record of all the thoughts I've had in response to my stroke. As soon as I wake I thank my lucky stars I'm alive and thinking. I'm thankful for the fact that I have thoughts at all. But there is no way every little detail that comes to mind, every recollection, will be saved. If only I could press a "save" key and select what I consider memorable. But then, I tell myself, you know nothing is permanent. Be happy. Perhaps I'm returning to normal and the filters are working once more.

Embrace the tree! Embrace the breath! Embrace the morning song of birds welcoming the rising sun. The world is a magical place and the brain, well, the brain is an extraordinary world in itself.

August 30, 2013. And here I am again saddened by the loss of another great writer, the Irish poet and Nobel laureate, Seamus Heaney.

For some reason I am taking these losses personally.

Heaney, too, suffered a stroke, a few years earlier, in 2006. I don't know if his stroke had anything to do with his death. Apparently the evening before he died he collapsed outside a Dublin restaurant. I recall my fall on the golf course a few weeks before I suffered my stroke. A moment of darkness. And I wonder if there is a connection; if this is what he experienced.

I worry about my own future, about what surprise is in store for me.

Strokes leave you feeling so vulnerable or as Heaney himself remarked, "babyish." His poems in *Human Chain*, published in 2010, dwell in part in that painful and exposed place that strokes open in the heart. His friend Colm Tóibín described *Human Chain* as "his best single volume for many years, and one that contains some of the best poems he has written . . . a book of shades and memories, of things whispered, of journeys into the underworld, of elegies and translations, of echoes and silences."

Stroke talk.

I first read and studied Heaney's poems at Leeds, shortly after *Death of a Naturalist* had been published. What remarkable poems. We met when he came to read at the University of British Columbia in 1970 or '71. I can't recall if it was the fall or spring of that academic year. With his permission I made a tape of his reading. He sang with such incantatory power; his poems, filled with enchantment and wisdom, ran in the blood. His language inhabited his home place intimately; his grief was haunting. His brilliance had something to do with the way he looked at everyday things.

Strokes show no discrimination.

Hearing about writers who have died of stroke is not the way I want to reconnect with the literary world.

Over time, the gaps in my stroke narrative are increasing. I see these longer stretches of silence as a sign that I'm healing, as a signal of increasing emotional stability. Of peace and hope. Of less fear. I don't know why this is the case, but I still struggle with making decisions, which is frustrating for everyone around me. Usually there is nothing complicated about the choices I'm offered; I simply prefer to ramble about the countryside of my own thoughts.

October 11, 2013. I woke up this morning at 5:12 a.m. and quickly realized I felt as good as I've felt since having my stroke eleven months ago. This is the second time in two weeks I've felt this way. Almost normal, except for my arm which still refuses to behave and operate the way it's supposed to. I went to bed at eleven and fell asleep immediately. Consequently I had six hours of uninterrupted sleep. This is the only thing I can think of that those two days share in common. An extended period of uninterrupted sleep. Clearly the brain and body need rest. I've known this for some time. Every one of my caregivers and therapists has repeated this piece of advice over and over, but sometimes what you know to be good for you is difficult to achieve. Sometimes temptation gets in the way, other times it's bloody-mindedness and determination that push recovery, and sometimes it's pain and your body struggling against your will. What doesn't feel right takes over and has you doing things that are at odds with your recovery.

Imagine how I'd feel with a full eight hours of uninterrupted sleep.

But now I know how valuable rest is; my body and brain keep telling me so. I feel energy throughout my being that's lacking when I sleep in fits and starts. I know this to be true, yet for the most part I have felt powerless to override the malaise that accompanies the brain attack. Perhaps this is something every stroke survivor experiences.

When I awoke, Virginia Woolf came to mind. What an extraordinary writer she was; what insight she had into human nature, into the human mind. What other great works would she have contributed to our story if she had lived a longer life? What would she, of all writers, have made of brain plasticity? And would knowledge of brain plasticity have helped her to deal with her own particular demons?

And then I thought about Alice Munro winning the Nobel Prize. And, I said to myself, it's about time. I had felt this way for many years, from the time I interviewed her for the Australian journal, *Meanjin*. When I phoned and asked her if she wanted to read the final manuscript of the interview she said: "No, just make me sound intelligent."

What do Virginia Woolf and Alice Munro share in common that they should slip into my mind at the same time? I'm in awe of the connections and associations the brain makes with such casual ease, as though thoughts are sharing a cup of coffee or going on a picnic together.

December 27, 2013. My granddaughter, Flora, along with her parents, my daughter Nicole and her husband Iain, came for Christmas dinner, a little over a month after the anniversary of my stroke. Upon their arrival I noticed that Flora was paying me much closer attention than she had on past visits. She circled about me like a spinning top, as if for a brief time I was the still-point of her cosmos.

When the two of us sat down at the table, she turned to her mother, and said: "Mommy, Poppa's hand is a lot better."

"Really?" I said, as I glanced at her with a certain degree of misgiving.

"Yes," she insisted without pause, and picked up her Minnie Mouse fork and began to eat.

I looked for a hint that she might be teasing me, although I don't think kids master this kind of deception at quite so young an age.

My granddaughter had earlier surprised me when she requested to sit beside me at the table. Before she sat down she had pushed her chair closer, so we were rubbing elbows.

I knew right away this was a gesture that brought us both mutual pleasure.

Initially, though, I was taken aback. My granddaughter is three and will turn four on January 2, 2014. When she had last seen me at Thanksgiving in October, she had been reluctant to give me a hug or let me touch her. I think she still associated me with my days in a wheelchair when I looked more like a Transformer figure than a grandparent. When I reached out to her, she would shy away from me with fairly unsubtle manoeuvres. Now she not only hugged me voluntarily, she sought out my attention and readily stroked my hand, which was like a kitten struggling to stand on its own. Something had changed.

That a three-year-old should notice such subtle changes seemed to me remarkable and heartening. What I have come to see as glacial movements I like to think she sees as a promise which I hope to keep — to watch her grow into a woman.

April 20, 2014. As I sat at my desk writing, I learned that Alistair MacLeod had died from complications of a stroke he had suffered in January. Aside from being a gifted writer, the most careful of craftsman, he was a gentle, kind soul. We first met in 1984 in Scotland where he was the Canadian-Scottish Exchange Writer. Throughout his reading in an Edinburgh pub he was editing his story, listening to every syllable as it rolled off his tongue.

He had a way of seeing, of giving voice to thoughts, images, passions, silences, experiences that sought refuge and understanding outside time. Outside the narrow confines of history. A stroke, I thought, might have robbed him of his expansiveness and generosity. And so much more.

I wanted to weep.

■

Although I know that a part of my brain has been killed off, I also know that the healthy part of my brain that has survived the onslaught has taken over and is trying to construct new pathways back to a version of who I was. Every so often I have these little epiphanies where a part of my brain says to me, "Ah, that's how you used to do it." I am amazed still when these occur; each one brings a small measure of recovery. I literally visualize something that I had forgotten or I assumed I was no longer capable of doing, and suddenly a muscle awakening or a nerve impulse refiring becomes a possibility.

Most recently this happened to me when I jogged a few feet while walking through the obstacle course my trainer, Scott de Búrca, had set up for me.

A graduate in Sports Science and Health from the Institute of Technology Tallaght in Dublin, Scott prefers the Celtic or Irish version of his name to the anglicized, Scott Burke. When he counts he says ". . . five, four, tree (the 'h' dropped), two, one." He's a joy to work with, short, nimble, and always on his toes, as if he's attempting some singular form of "step dancing." And he's cheeky, if not borderline mocking. Needless to say, we get along.

When we first met he told me he hoped to join the French Foreign Legion at some time in the future. Meanwhile, he has become a stepfather to two sons and a daughter, whom he talks about with such love that I know he'll never leave them. He's made an enduring pact with himself and with them that he'll want to keep.

After spending over a year rehabbing on my own, I hired Scott as my personal trainer. Immediately my recovery shifted gears.

Every session, he greets me with a handshake, testing my grip; and every session he asks me how I'm doing. Have I felt any new aches and pains since we last met, what kind of a day am I having, how is my mood, have I noticed any changes in strength and mobility, am I eating well enough, am I getting enough sleep?

"I want to know, so be honest with me," he says. "I want to know what's happening with you, so no bullshit. Give me the straight goods."

"I'm fine," I answer, hesitating. "For a man who's had a stroke."

Then I wave my cane at him.

"Don't be feeling sorry for yourself. There are lots worse off."

The first time he said this I was a little annoyed. Did he consider me dishonest or stupid? But when I turned to look at him I could see an impudent grin spread across his face.

"Give me five minutes on the bike," he replies, "and a few stretches. Then we'll get to work. It's important for you to warm up and to keep your muscles stretched. We want extension, not flexion. Atrophy is the biggest problem after a stroke, especially if you've been bedridden for any length of time. We don't want you wasting away, not that that's a likely problem with you," he says, eyeing me up and down as if I'm an old, baggy suit of clothes. "When you lose muscle memory your muscles tend to contract, a response in part to fatigue."

What I appreciate most about Scott is that he views what we're doing as a collaborative effort. He wants to know in which way a particular exercise is helping me. He agrees with me that balance is our sixth sense, so we have built this idea into all the walking drills. Arm exercises are simple. We use a six-foot length of two-inch dowelling material (a broom handle would work just as easily), and I push against him with both arms while he resists. Then he pushes against me while I resist. Then I pull, he resists; he pulls, I resist. At the end of each drill he pulls both of my arms towards him, maximizing extension. Stretching like this is pure bliss.

Then he brings coordination and my brain into the action. While I sit, we box. He uses focus mitts and I punch. As he moves the mitts around I have to track him. I'm amazed how quickly my brain has responded to following his movements. Each week we increase the speed and lately I have been doing this boxing exercise while standing.

Balancing.

Keeping everything we do in balance.

Since being released from hospital therapy my right hand has been a claw — almost a closed fist. I had taught myself to write, but I still couldn't spread my fingers. To increase extension Scott started to throw tennis balls towards my hand from a distance of about four feet. At first they hit my knuckles, bounced off my chest or head, or scooted on past me. Now I can follow and catch the ball and throw it back from a distance of ten to twelve feet. Initially, the degree of concentration it took to follow the ball was almost overwhelming, now it's becoming a habit. Releasing objects is more of a challenge. My fingers close when I attempt to throw the ball underhand and it goes straight up in the air, occasionally landing on my head. Scott finds this amusing and chortles.

"Good, very good, do you think you could do that again?"

But my brain is relearning.

The obstacle course was another matter. Another degree of difficulty — of recovery — conquered.

It consisted of a fifteen-foot ribboned ladder laid out on the floor, followed by five orange cones placed in a zigzag pattern, twenty feet between each cone, ending in a finishing line. The object was to step with both feet into each square that formed the ladder, out the other side, and into the next square with both feet, and out the opposite side. There were ten squares in total to navigate, the sort of routine football players undertake to improve their foot speed. Followed by a dash (in my case a laboured walk using my cane) around the cones.

On the first day that Scott set up the course, I walked through it three times, the first time in something like fifty-two seconds, the second time in thirty-six seconds. Gaining in confidence, I managed to lift and place my feet a little more quickly.

Towards the end of my third effort, Scott yelled out, "You're going to beat your last time, Ron. Hurry, I know you can do it."

Without a thought, as I turned the corner around the fourth cone, I carried my cane and lunged forward for about three or four steps.

"Twenty-eight point six seconds," Scott cheered.

The improved time meant nothing to me. But the sensation I felt in my brain, a form of jogging, was indescribable. Awesome, like a "big bang" going off in my head. It was a case of "recognizing" something innately, not merely remembering it. I felt it! I sensed myself jogging in my brain! Or, as my friend Edwin Webb suggested, "Perhaps you were imaging the brain activity itself — 'thinking the brain into thinking properly.'"

Perhaps I had experienced the forging of a new neural pathway.

Defiance.

Recovery seemed to me more like treading water and then mindfully swimming into the future.

I have always loved Joseph Conrad's metaphysical understanding of man's potential when he writes in *Heart of Darkness*, "The mind of man is capable of anything — because everything is in it, all the past as well as all the future."

The structural makeup of the human mind is under constant review and is the subject of ceaseless never-ending conjecture. The debate has really just begun and will likely continue for as long as we have thoughts. Crammed into our brains is approximately the same number of neurons as there are stars in the Milky Way, roughly one hundred billion of them — an unimaginable number. Each neuron receives input from tens of thousands of the other neurons and in turn sends messages to still tens of thousands of others, adding up to over one million-billion connections. The Nobel laureate, Gerald Edelman, in his book about the brain, *Bright Air, Brilliant Fire*, speculated that if you were to attempt counting the links, one per second, you might finish thirty-two million years later.

Equally mind-boggling numbers appear in Michio Kaku's *The Future of the Mind*. He proposes:

> You may have to travel twenty-four trillion miles, to the first star outside our solar system, to find an object as complex as what is sitting on your shoulders. The mind and the universe pose the greatest scientific challenge of all, but they share a curious relationship. On the one hand they are polar opposites. One is concerned with the vastness of outer space, where we encounter strange denizens like black holes, exploding stars, and colliding galaxies. The other is concerned with inner space, where we find our most intimate and private hopes and desires. The mind is no farther than our next thought, yet we are often clueless when asked to articulate and explain it. (2)

Here a proposition about travel into outer space turns into a voyage inside the brain. Even the most mundane tasks require sorting, prioritizing, organizing, and then a response so we can get on with our day. And the brain accomplishes all this in nanoseconds, with ease.

The brain weighs roughly three pounds and runs on the equivalent of between ten and twenty watts of power. Yet, according to experts, a computer as smart as the human brain would require at least ten megawatts of power, the amount of energy produced by a small hydroelectric plant.

But it's not just scientists who tell us about some of the challenges we face in understanding the brain. Bill Bryson in *A Short History of Nearly Everything* warns us, perhaps tongue-in-cheek, of some of the brain's limitations: "Brain cells last as long as you do. You are issued a hundred billion or so at birth, and that is all you are ever going to get. It has been estimated that you lose five hundred of them an hour, so if you have any serious thinking to do there really isn't a moment to waste." (373) After a stroke, or any other form of brain assault, this loss rises exponentially and is far too often catastrophic.

And yet only a few years after Bryson made this claim, his statement turned out to be untrue. Dr. Michael Hill says: "There are brain stem cells that do become new neurons in life and part of recovery is about making new neurons." Another reason for optimism!

As a kid I remember lying on the grass outside our family home and staring up into the night sky, trying to count the stars overhead. In no time at all I was on numerical overload as I drifted off into all sorts of fanciful speculations. I tried to close the immensity of my separation and distance from the stars by wondering if there was other life out there and by doing what had been done for millennia, picking out the shapes the stars formed.

One of my favourite stories, told in the Hindu tradition, contends that we are the dream of the god, Brahma. Perhaps each one of us is a cosmic entity. Maybe the neurons in our brains are the stars in someone else's universe. Perhaps when we look up into the night sky we are looking into another being's brain — a brain that is dreaming us.

What if we are beings living inside of beings, living inside of beings, like Matryoshka or Russian dolls?

If indeed we are living inside another being, then Hindu cosmology — one possible manifestation of this idea — provides a mathematical equation as complex as anything in modern physics. In *The Wonder That Was India* A.L. Basham explains that "the cosmos passes through cycles within cycles for all eternity. The basic cycle is the *kalpa*, a 'day of Brahma,' or 4,320 million earthly years. His night is of equal length." A combined day and night of Brahma equals 8.64 billion earthly years. While he lives, Brahma daily creates the universe and again re-absorbs it at night while he sleeps. In some traditions the process is reversed and Brahma creates the universe at night when he falls asleep and dreams our cosmos. When he wakes, creation dissolves only to be recreated anew when he falls asleep. In this view of the pulsating universe we live our lives within the dream of God. Or, put another way, we come alive when God dreams.

What do these mythologies and all this conjecture have to do with my rehabilitation as a stroke survivor? With therapists helping me to bend back into a familiar shape and into the individual I'd lost? With the person I was before the stroke and with the person I have become?

Perhaps nothing, at least not directly. Yet my ability to meditate, contemplate, and fantasize tells me I am recovering. My love of story shows me that once again I have a healthy brain.

When I was in the hospital I could hear a constant buzz about me, like bees to oregano. Rehab talk. But I was excluded from all occult medical discussions. The assumption was that after the brain attack I wouldn't understand.

Possibly.

That seems plausible enough.

Now I realize that after my stroke it's unlikely I'll return to be the person I once was, mentally or spiritually. I have both lost and gained things that define who I am as a person.

Yet the question still remains: Can I continue to rebuild? Reconstruct? Repair?

Well, yes . . . yes . . . I believe I can. Advances in treatment, therapy and our understanding of how the brain works continue to improve the outcomes of stroke.

Reading and thinking and yearning have brought me to a place where I believe anything is possible.

■

As ice blankets the ponds in front of the house, and this record of my stroke journey comes to a close, I'm reminded of a little village in the north of England, in Lancashire, near to where some dear friends of ours live. Downham, in the Ribble Valley, has to be one of the most idyllic villages in all of England, especially when a layer of hoar frost lies upon the hills. There is a small church, a graveyard, a tea shop, a bridge to cross, and talk of witches, not to mention sheep enclosed in fields surrounded by dry stone walls, all the makings for the marriage of the imagination and metaphor. When I think of this village at the bottom of Pendle Hill, I feel peace . . . and a quiet settles upon me.

ELEVEN

Recovery: Some Final Thoughts

Strokes teach their own lessons, lessons to do with pain, anger, fear, love and expectancy. Sharper than pain and blunter than fear, hope after a stroke toys with the mind.

How has my stroke changed me?

There are times when I weep for what Pat has had to endure. And yet, I know she would quarrel with my use of the word "endure." Our bones and flesh are entwined.

I now appreciate the importance of family and friends much more than I did before the stroke. Kindness, fragility, tenderness, laughter — these are the qualities I have come to admire most in the people around me. A Cooper's hawk landing in the fir tree outside Pat's study window, the scent of lavender rising from the terraces, a child's laughter as a swing climbs into the sky, a full moon filtered through alder branches, the first flower on my favourite camellia, the grunt of sea lions welcoming the herring run — these and much,

much else all delight me. Simple joys. My granddaughter grows and, even at the age of five, walks into the future with the confidence of a young woman. Her mother and father, both archaeologists, have taught her to listen to the stories of clam gardens, to appreciate the ancient tales told by the First Peoples of this coast. Those people who built stone walls along the shoreline to nurture clams, which would grow larger and more plentiful. Their harvest also included geoducks, mussels, oysters, sea cucumbers, kelp and small fish caught by the movement of the tides.

Post-stroke I have been awed by the breathtaking beauty of the planet, much more so than I was before I had my eyes opened by the bombing of my brain. I always took the world about me for granted; now I worry about its survival. Why, oh why, I wonder do we deny our role in climate change or global warming? I find our equivocation on the subject disturbing, and I mourn the erosion of the paradise in which we live.

Of known species how many will disappear from the planet in the next one hundred years, let alone the next millennium? "Extinct" is a word about which we have a reckless and cavalier attitude. Its meaning truly eludes us, hides behind a smokescreen of opportunity and privilege. We still allow trophy hunters with high-powered rifles to prey on grizzly bears in the rapidly shrinking habitat of the great Pacific Northwest rainforest. And if a bear or cougar or wolf crosses into "our" habitat, we "euthanize" it. Our pursuit of gratification consolidates our power as the masters of technology and feeds our sense of entitlement. Our quest for wealth and power seems even pettier, more destructive, than it did before. The violence we commit towards others, especially the increasing numbers forced to live in refugee camps and poverty, should cause us shame. Tyrants and murderers come in all shapes and disguises and they love to build bigger and higher walls.

Who's suffered the brain attack, I wonder?

Probably the most important thing I've learned is that I need far less stress in my life. That's why I'm writing this note to myself at 4:32 in the morning. An idea popped into my head, something that I thought was important, and I crawled out of bed to make sure it wasn't lost in the hills and valleys of some unfamiliar dreamscape. I stumbled to my computer and typed down the following. Actually I still peck with one finger.

This morning I was lying in bed thinking that my greatest hope for the future of our species is that we will realize that the three pounds that sit on top of our neck and shoulders is a far more interesting "device" to explore than the digital versions we carry in our pockets or backpacks. We are so easily distracted by the trivial, superficial and, ultimately, inconsequential. Everywhere these days I see people engaged and engrossed with a tiny screen, their thumbs tapping away robotically.

What has this done to our imaginations, to our ability to daydream? With all the research that is being carried out these days on the brain, we should be realizing that our own brains are the most exciting playgrounds for exploration in the universe. Perhaps schools and universities will once again recognize this fact and start doing what they should have been doing all along: teaching people the importance of thought, what we used to teach in the disciplines of philosophy, history and the language of the place where we live. What at one time was the function of story.

It's all well and good to train people to perform certain tasks, but it is equally important to emphasize that they do so thoughtfully. We have lost our way. We no longer value the quality of our thinking.

A while ago, a friend phoned to ask how I was doing. She is an intelligent, well-informed person, a fine writer and a successful career woman. I told her that my recovery was continuing but that it was a slow process. She expressed some degree of surprise; she thought I would be fully recovered by now. "Hasn't it been well over a year since the event?" she asked.

"Yes," I said to the timeline, "but, no," I explained, "I believe my recovery will continue, but I doubt that I'll ever reach full recovery."

Again she expressed surprise. She told me that it was her understanding that if a stroke didn't kill you, full recovery was inevitable.

"No," I said, "only change is inevitable. Strokes are the major cause of disability amongst people. Not only are there different types of strokes, but every one is different, as different as the individual brain to which it has happened. In my case, I was fortunate to survive with little damage to my cognitive abilities but my physical being was seriously compromised."

Let me end by stating what I believe to be a well-disguised, hence undisclosed, but self-evident truth: Unless you have experienced a stroke you can't begin to know what it's like. Even stroke experts, who I believe are doing extraordinary, cutting-edge research on the brain, can only guess what a stroke must feel like, can only speculate on the journey stroke patients take. And the more severe the stroke is, the greater the conjecture. This may be the only time when the old adage "until you've been there" actually applies. Having a stroke is unique. At least at this time in history, it is unparalleled as a human experience.

Wait just a minute, you will say, this is true of any illness, major or minor. Every malady known to man presents its own challenges. And I would have to concede that even for someone suffering from a hangnail, the pain can seem unbearable, the inconvenience intolerable. We become inconsolable when in pain. Put simply, suffering of any sort runs from unpleasant to life-changing; in the moment each seems as serious as the other. And invariably the suffering will be highly subjective.

A common cold in a toddler can be as upsetting, as disturbing, for a new mother as someone receiving news that they have a stage four cancer. Most of us have suffered from back pain — a lightning bolt down the sciatic nerve — which leaves us hobbling for days or weeks on end and eventually sends us to our bed for relief. Soon we discover nothing provides respite. No matter how we move or contort our body, the pain persists. And the best medical professionals can do, after they've experimented with various forms of body manipulation, injections, massage therapy, needles inserted along the body's meridians and drugs, is suggest we get some rest. Time will heal the problem, they tell us.

There are some illnesses for which I don't want to receive a diagnosis — ALS, Parkinson's, Alzheimer's, MS amongst those at the top of the list. But once you've received the diagnosis for any one of these illnesses, the prognosis can be relatively clear-cut. The blueprint is fairly predictable. Each has a distinct pathology. And treatments, while being constantly reviewed and updated — not quickly enough when I consider military spending and the indulgences the wealthy lavish on themselves — usually follow a pretty strict protocol. We have an increasingly broadening understanding of how the body works. Daily discoveries add to our knowledge.

But when part of the brain is killed off we still face an insurmountable mystery.

Thoughts, emotions and memories are invisible.

Stroke protocols are limited.

Happily, a new, highly successful stroke treatment was recently reported on in national and international media — endovascular thrombectomy — where a neuro interventional radiologist or surgeon within hours of a stroke's onset inserts a thin tube into an artery of the groin and then guides it by X-ray imaging to the site of the blockage in the brain. A retrievable stent is then deployed to ensnare the blood clot and restore blood flow to the brain.

In a news release, Dr. Michael Hill has said, "These results will impact stroke care around the world." Dr. Hill is a senior author of the study and a professor at the University of Calgary's Cumming School of Medicine, one of the foremost stroke research centres in the world.

Within a few years, this life-saving, life-changing procedure might be as commonplace as the various heart attack protocols. While we still won't know what's happening in the mind, we'll be able to limit the damage a stroke can do and the misery it can cause.

More and more patients will walk away unencumbered from their strokes.

My recovery, even to me, moves slowly and remains almost imperceptible. Yet I know recovery never ends and the rate at which it happens is totally unpredictable.

The Icelandic writer, Sjón, in his novel *The Blue Fox*, has one of his characters quote Ovid, twice: "All things change — nothing perishes." And later: "The burden that is well borne becomes light." This is good advice for anyone who is willing to listen but more so for the stroke survivor struggling with her or his doubts about recovery. And those doubts, I learned, are inevitable.

Such is our appetite for life.

Indeed, nothing perishes.

An old Irish proverb says: "When God made time He made plenty of it."

My right arm and hand have been the last parts of me to show signs of recovery. Even now, two years after the stroke, at the time of this writing, I notice daily miniscule changes. Slow, almost immeasurable changes — like watching a narcissus bulb in spring growing towards the sun — but changes nonetheless. I have become accustomed to the slowness of recovery, something that in the beginning caused me considerable frustration. I wanted everything to happen yesterday, as my mother used to say about me when I was a kid growing up. If nothing else, the stroke has taught me patience.

So now, as I say, expect change, it's inevitable.

Writing this stroke memoir has given me reason for optimism. When I jot down the occasional note I hold my pen as if it were a quill or a brush used in calligraphy. I imagine that I'm capable of creating fine tapered lines and curls with a single stroke (that word again) rather than meaningless blotches. I'm confident that with time I will be liberated from the erratic spasms and the daily pain. For the time being, though, when I'm swimming or exercising in the pool, everything stops hurting. That's when I know for certain that from this point on any level of recovery is a blessing; another chance to love and to be loved in this world.

Ron Smith
March 2015

■ ■ ■ SELECT BIBLIOGRAPHY

Barnes, Julian. *Levels of Life*. Toronto: Vintage Canada Editions, 2013.

Basham, A.L. *The Wonder That Was India*. New York: Grove Press, 1954.

Bauby, Jean-Dominique. *The Diving Bell and the Butterfly*. New York: Harper Perennial, 2008.

Berger, John. *Here Is Where We Meet*. London: Bloomsbury, 2005.

Berger, John. *Keeping a Rendezvous*. New York: Pantheon, 1991.

Bryson, Bill. *A Short History of Nearly Everything*. Toronto: Random House, 2004.

Conrad, Joseph. *Heart of Darkness*. New York: W.W. Norton & Co., 1963.

Cummings, E.E. *Poems: 1923–1954*. New York: Harcourt, Brace & World, 1954.

Doidge, Norman. *The Brain That Changes Itself*. New York: Penguin, 2007.

Doidge, Norman. *The Brain's Way of Healing*. New York: Viking, 2015.

Edelman, Gerald. *Bright Air, Brilliant Fire*. New York: Basic Books, 1993.

Foer, Joshua. *Moonwalking with Einstein*. New York: Penguin, 2011.

Genova, Lisa. *Left Neglected*. New York: Gallery Books/Simon & Schuster, 2011.

Hanh, Thich Nhat. *No Death, No Fear*. New York: Riverhead Books, 2002.

Hemingway, Ernest. *The Old Man and the Sea*. New York: Charles Scribner's Sons, 1952.

Hobson, J. Allan. "Sleep and dream suppression following a lateral medullary infarct: a first-person account." *Consciousness and Cognition* 11, 377–390. Laboratory of Neurophysiology, Massachusetts Mental Health Center, Harvard Medical School, 2002. Available online at www.sciencedirect.com.

Hui-Yan, Chi & Carl Stimson. *Stroke: Help from Chinese Medicine*. Beijing: People's Medical Publishing House, 2011.

Joseph, Eve. *In the Slender Margin*. Toronto: HarperCollins, 2014.

Kaku, Michio. *The Future of the Mind*. New York: Doubleday, 2014.

Klein, Bonnie Sherr. *Out of the Blue: One Woman's Story of Stroke, Love and Survival*. Berkeley, CA: Wildcat Canyon Press, 1997.

Lane, Patrick. *There Is a Season*. Toronto: McClelland & Stewart, 2004.

Maltz, Maxwell. *The New Psycho-Cybernetics*. New York: Prentice Hall, 2002.

Mayes, Frances. *Bella Tuscany*. New York: Broadway, 1999.

Mayes, Frances. *Every Day in Tuscany*. New York: Broadway, 2010.

McCrum, Robert. *My Year Off: Rediscovering Life after a Stroke*. Toronto: Knopf Canada, 1998.

Milne, A.A. *The World of Pooh*. Toronto: McClelland & Stewart, 1957.

Perlmutter, David. *Grain Brain*. New York: Little, Brown and Company, 2013.

Sacks, Oliver. *The Man Who Mistook His Wife for a Hat*. New York: Touchstone Edition, Simon & Schuster, 1998.

Selhub, Eva M. & Alan C. Logan. *Your Brain on Nature: The Science of Nature's Influence on Your Health, Happiness and Vitality*. Toronto: John Wiley & Sons Canada, 2012.

Shlain, Leonard. *The Alphabet Versus the Goddess*. New York: Viking, 1998.

Sjón. *The Blue Fox*. New York: Farrar, Straus and Giroux, 2008.

Taylor, Jill Bolte. *My Stroke of Insight*. New York: Viking, 2008.

Watt, Douglas F. "Commentary on Professor Hobson's first-person account of a lateral medullary stroke (CVA): Affirmative action for the brainstem in consciousness studies?" *Consciousness and Cognition* 11, 391–395. Quincy Medical Center, Boston University School of Medicine, 2002. Available online at www.sciencedirect.com.

■ ■ ■ ACKNOWLEDGEMENTS

Surviving a stroke is never a solitary affair, although, at times, as the victim of a brain assault, you feel as though you have departed the planet to follow a new orbit on another world. Those who were there in the early days after my stroke will know who they are and accept my gratitude. They made me feel lucky and blessed. As I say, my mind was often somewhere else, struggling with another mission — survival and recovery.

First and foremost, I owe my life to Dr. Thomas Dorran for his compassion and dedication to his oath as a healer. And I'm forever indebted to the emergency room staff at the Nanaimo Regional General Hospital for their quick and decisive response and action.

I'm grateful to all the staff in acute care and in the rehab unit — nurses, kitchen staff, volunteers, cleaning staff, therapists, technicians — and to my family, friends and neighbours — everyone who encouraged and helped with my care and recovery.

My thanks to Bill and Elaine Coleman, Keith Harrison, Kieran and Pattie Kealy, Gary Geddes and Ann Eriksson, Barb and Garnet Hunt, Dr. Bernie and Dr. Elaine Binns, Ted and Barb Simpson, Basil and Pauline Yelland, Gerry and Marg James, Peter Brooks, Bruce and Caryl Wiley, Bob Gillespie, Faye and Joe Rosenblatt, Randal Macnair, Linda Murdoch, Barrie and Karen Philp, Brian and Barb Philp, Guy Philp and Frances Kern; all helped see me through the early struggle.

Thanks also to Brian and Hazel Barnes and Nicoletta Barbarito for their long-distance concern.

Dr. Marius Styne, Elaine Murphy, Lisa Watson, Scott de Búrca, George and Liz Holmes, and the crew at the Fairwinds Recreation Centre all helped with my rehabilitation.

Dr. Claire Sira guided me to the work of Dr. Alan Hobson and Dr. Douglas F. Watt.

My thanks to Margaret Reynolds who put me in touch with Sally Harding, one of the principals in the Cooke Agency, who in turn guided me to Suzanne Brandreth who became my agent and who never wavered in her support for me or my book. Her counsel was always wise.

Early readers included Dr. Bob Prosser, Carol Matthews, Dr. Michael Hill, Bruce Hunter, Jean Woo, Liz Takac, Stephanie Lawrence, Dr. Glen Tibbits, Bill Murdoch and Merna Summers. Thank you everyone for your helpful comments and insights. Special thanks to Linda Ferron, Noreen Kamal and Pam Aikman Ramsay for tirelessly listening and contributing to "stroke talk" and for reading early versions of the text.

The group at the Heart and Stroke Foundation embraced Pat and me as members of their family. The work they do and the research they arrange and support is critical to advancement in stroke prevention and treatment. Research is the backbone of what the Heart and Stroke Foundation does. They need our support, now more than ever.

Thanks, also, to the Oceanside Stroke Recovery Group and the Stroke Recovery Association of BC.

To Katie White and Cheryl Mitchell of Stroke BC, Dr. Jill Cameron from the University of Toronto, and to all the dedicated therapists who attended and included me in their SSBC Stroke Rehab Collaborative, many thanks.

My correspondence with Dr. Richard Allen and with Dr. Allan Hobson was invaluable.

My thanks to Gillian McMillan whose blog led me to the wonderful cover image for *The Defiant Mind* by Jack Shadbolt.

I am grateful to Simon Fraser University for the use of the painting by Jack Shadbolt, "Bursting Orb," 1991, acrylic on canvas, 124.5 x 124.5 cm. Gift of Simon Fraser University via the Estate of Doris Shadbolt. City of Burnaby Permanent Art Collection. Courtesy Simon Fraser University Galleries, Burnaby, BC.

My gratitude to Ron Hatch, an old friend, and his editorial and design team, led by Meagan and Julie at Ronsdale Press, for showing so much care in publishing *The Defiant Mind*. Ron was willing to take the risk.

Ian and Virginia Garrioch not only assisted me with their reading and understanding of the manuscript, but they helped sustain Pat and me with food, talk and steadfast friendship.

Ada Donati, Edwin and Mary Webb, and Bill and Peggy New were constant companions through the writing process. Bill edited, with the help of "Red" (Peggy often encouraged), every paragraph, sentence and word. His care and passion for the written word are infectious. He/they all inspired.

From the very early days after my stroke, my daughter, Nicole, and son, Owen, (and their partners, Iain and Jen respectively, and my grand-daughter, Flora) were there by my side. Their support and love made the healing process much, much easier.

Finally, and always first, Pat has been a constant in whatever universe I have found myself inhabiting. She listened to me read each and every page over two long years. Her encouragement, emotional and intellectual support, and love have made my recovery and this book possible.

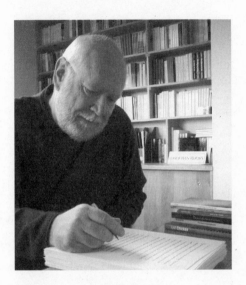

Ron Smith, born and raised in Vancouver, BC, is the author and editor of several books. For close to forty years he taught at universities in Canada, Italy, the States and the UK. In 2002 he received an honorary doctorate from the University of British Columbia and in 2005 he was the inaugural Fulbright Chair in Creative Writing at Arizona State University. In 2011 he was awarded the Gray Campbell Award for distinguished service to the BC publishing industry where he has played an essential role in the growth of literary, historical and public policy publishing. He lives with his wife, Patricia Jean Smith, also a writer, in Nanoose Bay on Vancouver Island.